How To Get Started With DIY Skincare

Abdullahi .F Broughton

All rights reserved. Copyright © 2023 Abdullahi .F Broughton

COPYRIGHT © 2023 Abdullahi .F Broughton

All rights reserved.

No part of this book must be reproduced, stored in a retrieval system, or shared by any means, electronic, mechanical, photocopying, recording, or otherwise, without written permission from the publisher.

Every precaution has been taken in the preparation of this book; still the publisher and author assume no responsibility for errors or omissions. Nor do they assume any liability for damages resulting from the use of the information contained herein.

Legal Notice:

This book is copyright protected and is only meant for your individual use. You are not allowed to amend, distribute, sell, use, quote or paraphrase any of its part without the written consent of the author or publisher.

Introduction

This is a comprehensive guide that empowers readers to take charge of their skincare routine by creating organic and homemade skin care products. The guide covers various aspects of skincare and provides practical advice on crafting effective and nourishing products for different skin types.

The guide begins with an introduction to the importance of skincare and the benefits it offers. It emphasizes the advantages of using organic and homemade skincare products, highlighting their natural and chemical-free qualities.

Readers are introduced to the basics of skincare, including different types of skin and how to identify their specific skin type using a helpful quiz. Understanding one's skin type is crucial for selecting the most suitable skincare products.

The guide dives into the world of DIY organic cleansers and toners, explaining the difference between these products and how to select and use them according to one's skin type. It provides readers with a variety of homemade recipes for cleansers and toners, allowing them to customize their skincare routine.

Moisturizers and face creams are explored in detail, with guidance on selecting the right products for different skin types. The guide offers readers a range of organic DIY recipes for moisturizers and face creams, empowering them to tailor their skincare products to their specific needs.

Eye creams, natural scrubs for the face and body, serums, and masks are also covered, providing readers with insights into the benefits of each product and step-by-step instructions on creating them at home. The guide includes recipes for various skincare products, allowing readers to experiment and find what works best for their skin.

The importance of proper storage and labeling of homemade skincare products is highlighted, along with considerations for gifting these goodies to friends and family.

The guide includes valuable information on ingredient dictionaries, explaining the uses of oils and other key skincare ingredients. It also clarifies skincare jargon, making it easier for readers to understand the world of natural skincare.

In summary, this book is a comprehensive resource that equips readers with the knowledge and skills to create their organic skincare products. It emphasizes the benefits of organic skincare, provides practical guidance on identifying skin types, and offers a wide range of DIY recipes for various skincare products, making it a valuable resource for those seeking a natural and personalized approach to skincare.

Contents

Chapter 1: Skin Care Basics 1
    The Importance of Skin Care 2
    Benefits of Skin Care 3
    Understanding Basic Skin Care Products 5
    Organic Skin Care 7
    Benefits of Using Organic Homemade Skin Care Products 8
    General Characteristics of Each Skin Type 10
    Identify Your Skin Type 12
    Take this Quiz to Identify Your Skin Type! 13

Chapter 2: DIY Organic Cleansers and Toners 16
    The Difference between Cleansers and Toners 17
    Selecting a Cleanser for Your Skin Type 19
    How to Use a Cleanser 20
    DIY Recipes for Organic Cleansers 21
    Toners 27
    Best Toners for Different Skin Types 28
    DIY Organic Toner Recipes 30

Chapter 3: Moisturizers and Face Creams 37
    Moisturizers 39
    Moisturizers for Different Skin Types 40
    DIY Organic Recipes for Moisturizers 42
    Face Creams 47
    Face Creams for Different Skin Types 48
    Organic DIY Recipes for Face Creams 50

  Eye Creams 54

Chapter 4: Natural Scrubs for Your Face and Body 56
  What Is a Scrub? 57
  Face Scrub vs. Body Scrub 59
  Facial Scrubs 60
  Types of Facial Scrubs for Different Skin Types 61
  DIY Organic Recipes for Facial Scrubs 62
  Body Scrubs 68
  Body Scrubs for Different Skin Types 69
  DIY Organic Body Scrub Recipes 70

Chapter 5: Serums and Masks 76
  Difference between a Mask and a Serum 77
  Face Serums 78
  Serums for Different Skin Issues 79
  Eye Creams 80
  How to Use a Serum in Your Skin Care Regime 81
  DIY Face Serum Recipes 82
  Face Masks 84
  Benefits of Using a Face Mask 86
  Masks for Different Skin Ailments 87
  Some Common Ingredients Used for Masks 92
  Important Considerations While Using Serums and Face Masks 94
  Shelf Life of DIY Skin Care Products 95

Chapter 6: Yummy Body Butters 96
  Body Butters with Specific Properties 105
  Different Types of Body Butters to Try Out 110
  Considerations before Using a Body Butter 111

Chapter 7: Organic Lotions and Balms 112
- Difference between Lotions and Other Creams and Moisturizers 113
- Lotions 115
- DIY Organic Lotion Recipes 117
- Shelf Life of Homemade Lotions 120
- Skin Balms 121
- Benefits of Using a Face Balm 122

Chapter 8: Labeling and Gifting Your Goodies 130
- Choosing the Container Material 132
- How to Store Homemade Cosmetics 134
- International Cosmetics Laws 140

Chapter 9: Ingredients Dictionary 143
- List of Oils and Their Uses 144
- All Other Ingredients 150
- Skin Care Jargon, Explained 155

Conclusion 184

Chapter 1: Skin Care Basics

The skin is the largest organ of our body and one of the most visible. It is a living barrier that protects us from the extremities of the outside world. This first chapter will teach you what skin care products are and why they are so important in our modern pollution-laden lives. We will then look at organic homemade skincare products to see how they compare to store-bought ones and explain their benefits and limitations. Finally, we will introduce you to a short quiz to identify your skin type and learn more about it!

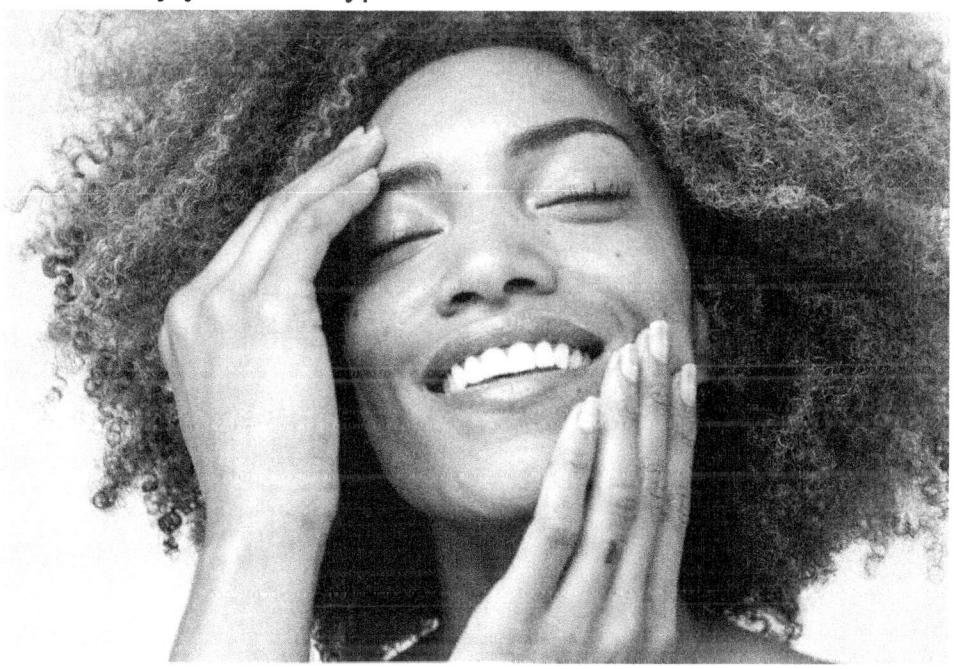

The Importance of Skin Care

Skin care is not just about looking good. It may be hard to believe, but your skin tells a lot about how well you take care of yourself and whether or not you practice proper hygiene. Your face can show what kind of health issues may lie beneath the surface. Therefore, it's essential to recognize these issues before they become a serious complication. This is where skin care comes in.

Ignoring the importance of skin care is something that many people do. If you do not take care of your skin, many things can go wrong. Some of the side-effects of ignoring skin care could be acne, dull skin, uneven skin tone, texture, and visible signs of aging. However, all of these can be prevented by incorporating appropriate skin care routines and habits into your life, which is why it's important to make sure you're doing everything right.

Your skin needs to be taken care of properly and hygienically to prevent numerous health issues.

Skin care may seem daunting at first, but it becomes second nature once you get into a routine, leading to an overall healthier lifestyle. Skin care is a great start to getting into the habit of taking care of yourself.

Benefits of Skin Care

The benefits of skin care are not just about looking good. Skin care is an integral part of your health and well-being. It can help you detect problems early so that they do not become worse in the future, which saves time, money, and pain in the long run.

Following a proper skin care regime offers the following benefits:

Improved Skin Tone, Texture, and Elasticity

This means that you can help delay signs of aging, such as wrinkles. Skin care also helps improve the health and condition of your skin by increasing blood circulation to promote fresh new cells (that will make up for dead or damaged cells, which are an inevitable part of life).

Enhanced Ability to Fight Infection

When taking care of your skin, it's crucial to protect it from the elements but also from harmful bacteria. This is especially important for skin that has been damaged by sunburn or wear and tear over time.

Protection against the Sun's Harmful Rays

No matter how young or old your skin is, the sun's ultraviolet rays can damage it. UVA and UVB rays cause signs of aging like wrinkles, age spots (also known as liver spots), sagging of the skin, leathering of the skin (a condition caused by loss of collagen where you see bunch-like folds in areas such as the elbows, knees, knuckles, and toes), along with skin cancer.

Protecting your skin from sun damage is one of the best things that you can do to protect yourself from all types of harmful effects. Even if it's cloudy outside or you don't feel direct sunlight on your face, UVA rays can penetrate through the clouds and thin layers of clothing.

Prevention of Wrinkles and Fine Lines

Prevention is the best way to keep wrinkles and fine lines at bay. As we age, our skin loses its elasticity and firmness, which causes it to sag and wrinkle over time. The earlier you start incorporating proper skin care habits, the better off your skin will be in terms of wrinkles and overall health. Your daily routine – such as wearing sunscreen (even when it's raining or snowing), washing your face with a gentle cleanser, and wearing moisturizer to prevent free radical damage – all go toward helping keep your skin healthy.

Reduced Appearance of Pores

Numerous factors such as pollution, smoking, poor diet, and stress can cause your skin to have a rough texture. Pores become more prominent over time due to the accumulation of dead skin cells that clog up the pores, creating blackheads or whiteheads. If left untreated, it can lead to acne breakouts. However, by taking care of your skin regularly, you can help reduce pores' appearance and prevent acne breakouts.

Reduction of Acne Breakouts

This is especially important for teenagers and young adults prone to acne breakouts. By washing with a gentle cleanser (not soap) daily, using moisturizer, practicing proper hygiene habits, including removing makeup before going to bed, you can help reduce the appearance of acne breakouts over time.

Thus, we see that skin care is an important part of everyone's health and well-being. Proper skin care can help you look younger, eliminate the need for expensive surgery or anti-aging creams, protect against harmful rays from the sun (UV), and prevent acne breakouts in both men and women. It also helps reduce fine lines, wrinkles, and pore size.

Understanding Basic Skin Care Products

There are numerous skin care products available on the market these days, specific to each skin type and issue. It's crucial to have good knowledge and expertise when selecting products to get the best results from your skin care regime.

Moisturizer

Moisturizer should be used regularly for normal, dry, or mature skin types as well as oily acne-prone skin types. It helps to maintain your skin's moisture levels, which makes you look more youthful and firmer by reducing fine lines, wrinkles, and pore size over time.

Sunscreen/Sun Protection Factor (SPF)

Sunscreen is an absolute must if you are going to be spending time outdoors. It helps protect the skin by blocking harmful UV rays, which can cause premature aging effects and can also lead to cancer in extreme cases. Wearing sunscreen every day will help reduce fine lines, wrinkles, and age spots while protecting your skin from sun damage.

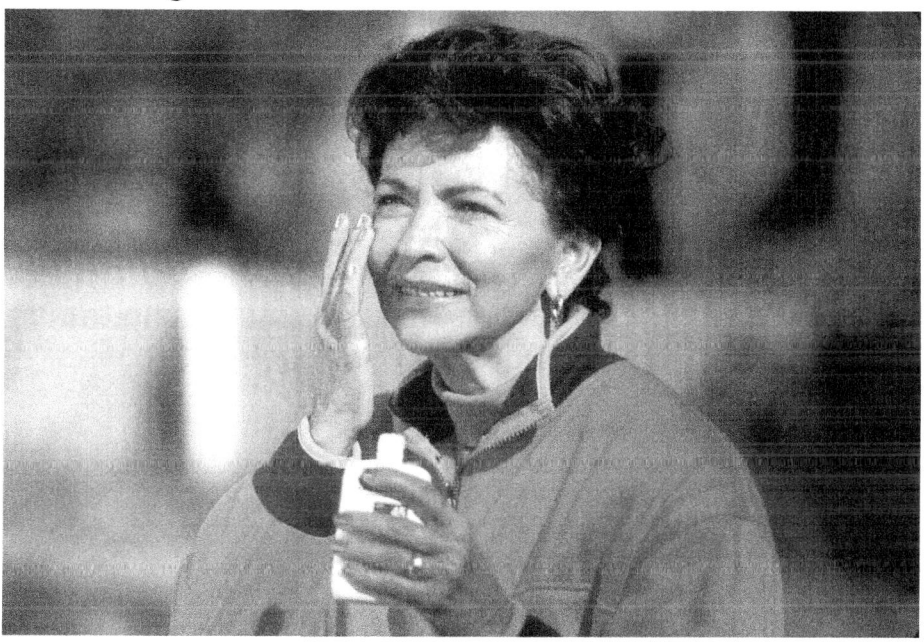

Cleanser

A gentle cleanser should be used to clean your skin and remove dirt, oil, bacteria, and makeup. Washing your face regularly with a mild cleanser helps protect the skin by eliminating harmful toxins that can lead to breakouts. It also helps reduce pore size and prevent acne breakouts.

Scrub

Scrubs can be used two to three times a week to remove dead skin cells and to keep your skin looking clear, smooth, and polished. Scrubbing helps reduce pores' appearance by removing excess dirt buildup on the skin surface. It also enhances blood circulation, which reduces acne breakouts over time.

Eye Creams or Serums

For those who are concerned about dark circles, puffiness, and fine lines around the eyes, eye creams or serums can be used to help reduce these symptoms. For best results, eye cream is applied daily in the morning and at night by gently patting it onto your skin in an upward motion towards your temple.

Mask/Exfoliating Mask

A mask should only be used once or twice a week to deep clean the skin. Masks are specifically designed for oily, normal, dry, or mature skin types and can help to reduce acne breakouts.

These are the basic types of skin care products available to everyone. Several specialized skin care products can be used if a person is concerned about pigmentation, anti-aging, and acne scarring. Still, everyone should start with these essential skin care items for the best results.

Organic Skin Care

Organic skin care is made with all-natural ingredients that are safe for your skin, but unlike "all-natural," to carry the "organic" label, such products are highly regulated, leaving you with less worry about harsh chemicals or toxins. This makes them even better for your skin – treating acne breakouts, reducing fine lines, wrinkles, and age spots. The main benefit of using organic skin care products is that they are often made with aloe vera, coconut oil, and shea butter – super skin nourishers!

All-natural skin care products can be much more expensive than their traditional counterparts. However, if you're concerned about harmful toxins in makeup or moisturizers, this is the way to go.

Many organic products can also be made at home by using ingredients that are 100% natural. This is a great way to save money while also having the satisfaction of knowing what's in your skin care products!

Benefits of Using Organic Homemade Skin Care Products

Using organic products is a great way to reduce the risk of developing skin cancer, age spots, wrinkles, and treating acne breakouts.

There are many benefits of using natural homemade skin care products, as shown below.

Saving Money

Store-bought organic skincare products can be expensive; however, making your own products at home can be a great way to save money. Homemade skin care items are also better for sensitive or acne-prone skin types because they don't contain harsh chemicals which irritate the skin over time.

All Natural Ingredients

Like using organic ingredients, all-natural ingredients pave the way to smooth, even skin. Instead of applying harmful toxins on the skin, organic products made with ingredients such as aloe vera nourish your skin while also protecting it from the sun.

Organic Skin Care Is Better for Your Skin

Many organic products can be made at home by using ingredients that are 100% natural. Synthetic products contain a lot of fillers and toxins, which can irritate your skin and cause unexpected breakouts. No chemicals, fertilizers, pesticides, or herbicides are used during the growing process of these products – and if the label says "organic," they have been closely regulated.

When you choose to go organic, you'll be using products that work in harmony with your skin and help you to maintain a healthy glow.

Health Benefits

Endocrine-disrupting chemicals such as sodium lauryl sulfate, parabens, and phthalates are present in many conventional skincare products. These chemicals can interfere with your body's hormones and cause cancer, diabetes, autism spectrum disorders (ASD), and Parkinson's disease. Such chemicals accumulate within the body and may cause health problems later in life.

Several studies show that chemicals in conventional skincare products can cause poor semen quality, infertility issues, and hormonal imbalances. The most significant concern is for pregnant women who use these products daily because they pass them on to their unborn children.

Environmentally Sustainable Products

One of the main concerns with using synthetic skincare products is that they are not environmentally sustainable. Many companies use toxic chemicals and other harmful ingredients during production, resulting in contamination of water sources, toxicity to local wildlife, and ground soil pollution. Organic products are sourced from natural ingredients that do not harm the environment in any way.

Organic products are better for wildlife and environmental health since they don't contain harsh chemicals, herbicides, or pesticides that alter soil quality over time. Many organic skincare brands use biodegradable packaging to reduce their environmental impact.

Making Organic Skin Care Products at Home

When you make organic skincare products at home, such as face cleansers and moisturizers, you can save money while still getting high-quality ingredients that promote healthy skin. You need to know which ingredients to use and how they work best for different skin problems. You can also brand these products and sell them (with the necessary approvals). Despite being handmade, these organic items must adhere to the same cosmetic rules and laws, and they should be packed and labeled appropriately, especially if you intend to offer your products for sale. We will discuss this in detail in chapter 8.

General Characteristics of Each Skin Type

There are several skin types; we'll discuss each one below.

Normal Skin

Normal skin is neither too dry nor too oily and has an even tone. It is resilient to environmental changes, such as temperature and humidity, therefore making your skin comfortable throughout the day. This type of skin doesn't have visible pores or blemishes. However, if you don't take care of this type of skin properly, you may experience breakouts and other issues.

Sensitive Skin

With sensitive skin, you are more susceptible to changes in the environment. This type of skin tends to be dryer than normal skin and has a thinner epidermis. It is prone to redness, irritation, rashes, or hives due to its lack of resilience when facing environmental factors like pollution or temperature fluctuations.

Dry Skin

Your skin is dry if it feels tight after washing your face or taking a shower. Additionally, the upper layers of the epidermis are filled with dead cells that make your complexion appear dull and flaky. Dryness can also cause red spots on your cheeks, making this type of skin prone to infections because it is more fragile.

Oily Skin

This skin type has more prominent pores than normal or dry skin, filled with oil and dead cells that accumulate in them. This type of skin gives off a shiny look no matter the temperature outside because its sebaceous glands produce more fluid than necessary for hydration balance. To counteract this type of skin, you should look for a powerful exfoliator and avoid applying heavy creams.

Combination Skin

This type is characterized by having both dry and oily spots on the face. One part of your complexion doesn't receive enough hydration while another gets too much oil. This causes blackheads to form faster than with other skin types.

Red Spots

The skin is more sensitive to sun rays and can get burned easily, leading your epidermis to produce pigments to protect itself from damage. This causes redness on the face, making you look older than you are because of how difficult it is for this type of skin to recover after being exposed to the sun.

Moles

Moles are small spots that can appear anywhere on the skin. They don't have a specific color, and they may darken over time due to hormonal changes, diet, or genetics. This skin is prone to having moles due to its irregular pigmentation.

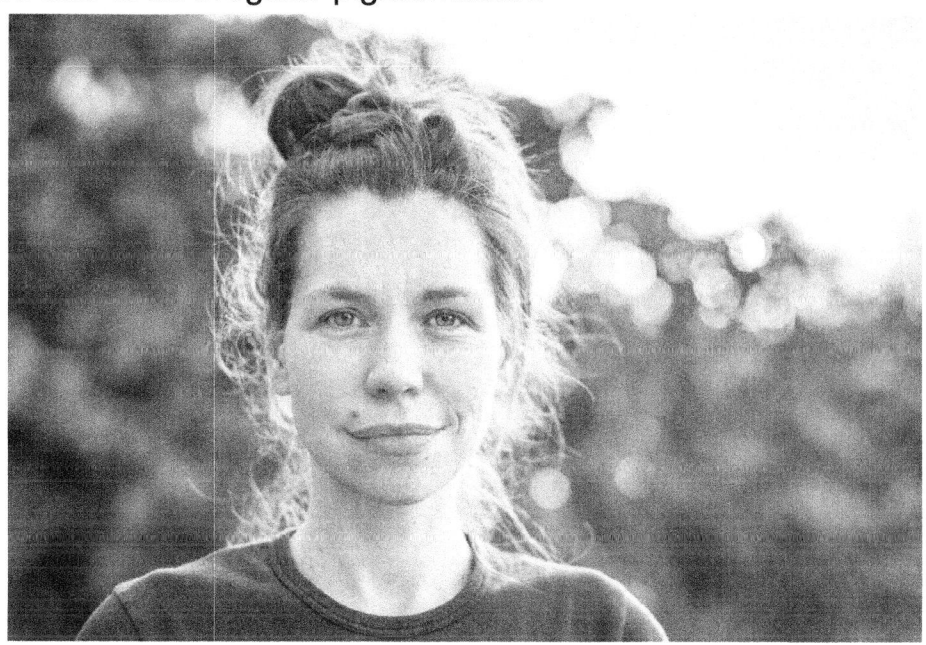

Identify Your Skin Type

You can identify your skin type by checking out these characteristics:

Normal Skin
- Comfortable and moist to the touch.
- It doesn't have visible pores or blemishes, but it may experience breakouts from time to time.

Sensitive Skin
- Soft with a thin epidermis which makes you more susceptible to changes in the environment.
- It is dry and tends to have red spots on your cheeks.

Dry Skin
- It feels tight after you've washed your face or taken a shower, which causes flaky skin that can lead to infections if not treated properly.

Oily Skin
- Has larger pores than normal skin.
- Produces more oil and dead cells that lead to blackheads forming faster than other skin types.

Combination Skin
- Can have dry or oily spots across your face at different times, which causes breakouts on some parts while others remain normal.
- This kind of skin tends to get red spots on the face more easily than other skin types because of its irregular pigmentation, making it difficult to recover after being exposed to the sun.

Red Spots
- They can appear anywhere on your body, but they are most common around the face.

Moles

- They are small spots that can appear anywhere on your body, but they are most common around the neck or face.

Take this Quiz to Identify Your Skin Type!

Here is a short quiz that can help you identify your skin type.

1. Which one of these statements best describes your facial pores?

    a. My facial pores are large and apparent all over my face.

    b. My pores are tiny and difficult to identify.

    c. My T-zone has moderate to large pores.

    d. My pores are visible, but they're really tiny.

2. How does your skin appear and feel when you wake up in the morning?

a. All of my skin is greasy and shiny.

b. My skin is yearning for moisture.

c. My eyes are swollen, and my skin is somewhat dehydrated.

d. My forehead is rather greasy, but my cheeks are extremely dehydrated.

e. My skin is lightly oiled all over.

3. At the end of the day, how does your skin appear and feel?

a. Crazy greasy. My makeup melts off my face, to be honest.

b. Just like the desert, I'm going to need moisturizer as soon as possible!

c. It's a bit dull and weary, mostly dry.

d. My skin is rarely oily at the end of the day.

4. How often does your skin break out?

a. Very Often

b. Never

c. I develop breakouts once a year due to climatic changes or stress.

d. Around my T-zone, I get a few pimples each month.

5. My preferred moisturizer is:

a. Light moisturizers irrespective of the season

b. Heavy moisturizers all year

c. In the winter, I use heavy moisturizers and light ones in the summer.

d. I use a specialized moisturizer, without which my skin breaks out.

6. Do you suffer from red, irritated, or flushed skin?

a. Yes – Especially after using new skincare products.

b. No – I don't get red, flush, or irritable skin very often.

7. Does your skin have evident sun damage?

a. Yes – my face is discolored and sun-damaged in many locations.

b. Yes, I have sun spots on my nose and cheeks.

c. No

8. The following is a must in my skincare routine:

a. Oil blotter

b. Rich moisturizer

c. Retinol

d. Calming mask

e. Toner

f. Exfoliating scrub

9. My greatest worry is...

a. I am concerned about Acne and flare-ups

b. Clogged pores and blackheads are my biggest worry

c. Patches of dry skin keep me up at night

d. The texture and tone of the skin are uneven

e. Fine lines and sunspots

f. A pimple or two here and there

Mostly As: Oily Skin

Mostly Bs: Dry Skin
Mostly Cs: Combination Skin
Mostly Ds: Sensitive Skin

We will look at each skin type in detail and the products you can use to treat them.

In this chapter, you learned all about how your skin type affects the health and appearance of your skin. If you want to take charge of what's going on with your skin, it may be helpful to identify which one of these four is your skin type: oily, dry, combination, or sensitive. Once you know that information, specific skincare products for each type can help address any issues and improve overall complexion.

Chapter 2: DIY Organic Cleansers and Toners

This chapter will explore different types of organic cleaners and toners specific to each skin type. We will also discuss why it's crucial for your skin to be balanced and how you can easily make these products at home!

The Difference between Cleansers and Toners

The primary distinction between a cleanser and a toner is that cleansers clean your skin. In contrast, toners help maintain the pH balance of your skin while also combating acne and dryness. A cleanser will remove dirt, oil, and makeup from the skin. Your face should feel clean after using a cleanser, but it shouldn't have that squeaky-clean feeling because cleaners do not deprive your skin of natural oils, which give protection against bacteria.

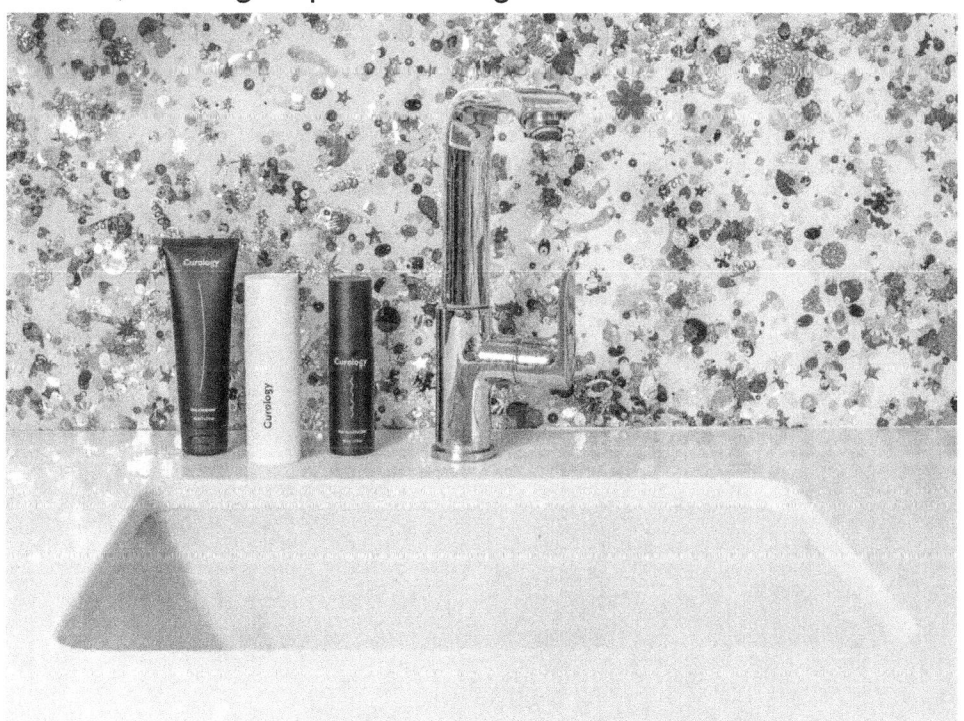

A toner will typically be dabbed all over the face with a cotton pad and helps close the pores after they've been opened up during cleansing. Toners control the pH by balancing the acidity of your skin. They're also great for eliminating any residual dirt and makeup that your cleanser may have missed. If you have a harsh cleanser, a toner will help remedy the dryness by adding extra hydration.

Cleansers

Cleansers are designed to remove impurities from the skin, such as sweat and dirt. They're often used before a moisturizer or serum is applied to help ensure that they have an easier time being absorbed into your pores. A cleanser should be strong enough to cleanse but mild enough not to irritate your skin.

Selecting a Cleanser for Your Skin Type

Normal Skin

Normal skin is neither dry nor oily, but it does require some additional care during winter to combat cold weather. You must choose a cleanser with moisturizing properties to keep your skin hydrated when temperatures drop. Look for ingredients like glycerin and olive oil, which will help draw moisture into your skin.

Sensitive Skin

If you have sensitive skin, look for a cleanser with anti-inflammatory ingredients like green tea extract or chamomile extract. These extracts are packed with antioxidants that can help prevent damage to your skin cells caused by free radicals in the environment and pollution. Also, steer clear of harsh chemicals that might trigger redness and irritation.

Acne-Prone Skin

If you have acne-prone skin, look for a cleanser with salicylic acid. This ingredient is known to unclog pores and prevent new ones from forming. Also, avoid ingredients like grapefruit seed extract, which can be too harsh on your delicate tissue.

Oily Skin

People who struggle with oily or shiny skin should opt for a cleanser that contains clay. Clay helps to soak up excess oil and reduces shine on your face without drying out your skin like other ingredients in harsh facial cleansers do.

Dry Skin

People with dry, sensitive skin should look for a gentle cleansing product with soothing organic aloe vera or coconut milk. These ingredients are known for their hydrating properties, which will help replace the moisture that your skin has lost.

How to Use a Cleanser

Using a face cleanser is quick and easy. Wet your face with warm water, then apply a small amount of cleanser on the area that needs treatment. Massage gently in circular motions for 30 seconds before rinsing thoroughly with cool water to close the pores. Remember to wash your hands before applying the cleanser to your face so you don't transfer germs or bacteria.

DIY Recipes for Organic Cleansers

Here are a few DIY recipes to get you started:

Honey Based Cleanser for Oily Skin

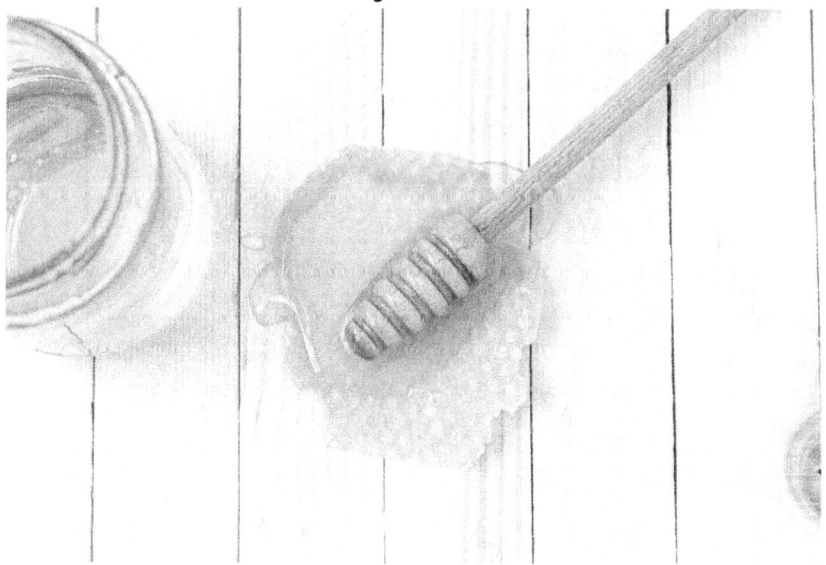

Raw and unpasteurized honey is beneficial in skin care. Using locally produced honey is highly recommended to promote wound healing, reduce pimples, increase moisture levels, soothe redness and inflammation, and minimize germs and sebum - without being overly harsh.

Ingredients:
- Avocado Oil - 1 Teaspoon
- Honey - 1/4th cup
- Essential Oil - 12 drops (use your favorite)
- Distilled Water - 1/4th cup
- Liquid Castile Soap - 2 tbs

Directions:

1. Take a jar and first mix water, soap, and honey gently together.

2. Make sure you stir gently to avoid foaming. If you have a soap dispenser handy, it is best to use it for this recipe.

3. Then add the avocado oil and the essential oils and mix all the ingredients thoroughly.

Expert Tip: *Add a pinch of baking soda to the mixture once in a while to use it as a scrub or an exfoliator. Take a little on your palm, mix in the baking soda, and gently apply it to your face. Use lavender or lemon oils if you are prone to acne!*

Lavender Oil Cleanser for Dry Skin

Lavender essential oil has anti-inflammatory and skin-loving properties, making it ideal for soothing irritation. This homemade cleaner is great when combined with moisturizing carrier oils such as grapeseed or sweet almond. You may use any of your favorite skin-friendly carrier oils in this recipe.

Expert Tip*: Stick to jojoba, grapeseed, or sweet almond oils. Olive oil is often impure and may cause inflammation when used on your face. Coconut oil may also be comedogenic, which causes more acne.*

Ingredients:
- 1 ounce of carrier oil (pick your favorite) (30 ml)
- 8 drops of lavender essential oil

Directions:
1. Fill a bottle halfway with a carrier oil.
2. Now add drops of lavender essential oil and mix everything together. This will create about an ounce (30ml) of product.

Caution:

If you've never used lavender essential oil on your skin, do a spot test on the inside of your wrist before applying the cleanser to your entire face. Using a washcloth or reusable cotton round wet with warm water, massage the oil into your skin. Repeat as needed to remove makeup by using wet cloth/reusable cotton round.

Oatmeal Cleanser for Sensitive Skin

When you have a sensitive skin type, look for a gentle cleanser to remove makeup and dirt. This recipe is perfect for you since oatmeal acts as a gentle exfoliator, removing dead skin cells to reveal maximum smoothness and soothing inflammation due to its anti-inflammatory properties.

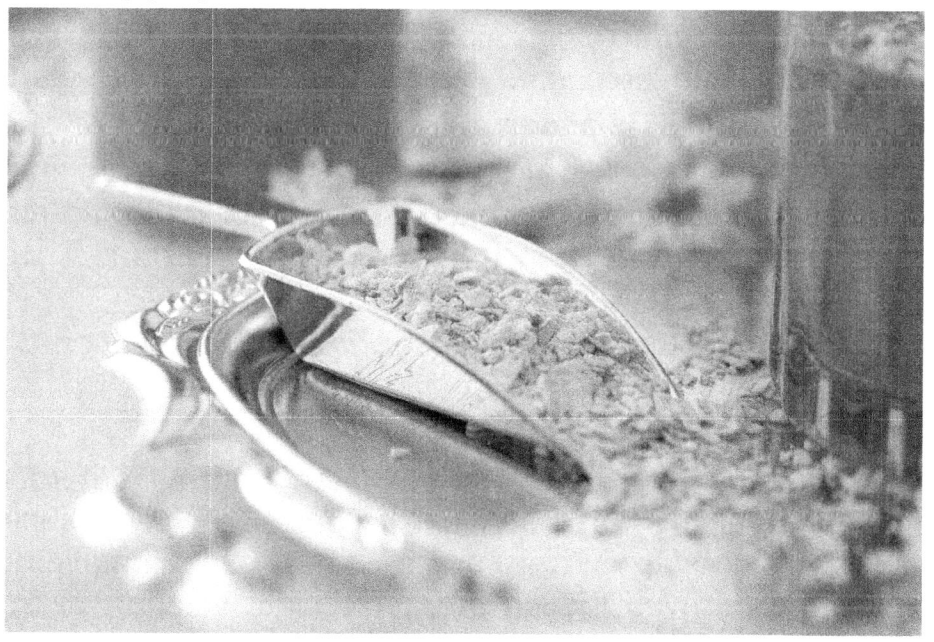

Expert Tip: *If you have oily or acne-prone skin, avoid using this cleanser at night because it can clog your pores.*

Ingredients:
- Rolled oats - 1/3rd cup (30 grams)
- Water - 1/2 cup (120 ml)
- Sugar or salt -1/4th teaspoon, finely ground, if possible. Use a pinch more for extra scrubbing effects. Do not use sea salts as they can irritate sensitive skin and cause inflammation.

Directions:
1. Mix all the ingredients in a bowl until you have a thick paste with no lumps remaining.

2. Use warm water, if needed, to help dissolve any oatmeal that is stuck together before applying it to your face.

3. Do not press too hard as it may aggravate your acne.

4. Rinse off the oatmeal with warm water and pat your face dry.

5. This recipe can be stored in an airtight container for two weeks when kept refrigerated, but it is best if used within a week of making the paste.

Apple Cider Vinegar Cleanser

Apple cider vinegar is acidic in nature and has antibacterial and anti-inflammatory properties. This makes it perfect for removing dirt, oil, and dead cells from your skin to reduce acne breakouts – without being too harsh on your face.

Expert Tip: *Do not store this cleanser. It has to be prepared fresh for every use.*

Ingredients:

- Water- 1/4 cup - Use distilled water if you have hard water or tap water high in impurities. If your skin type is sensitive, avoid using tap water as it can cause irritation and inflammation even though the apple cider vinegar will soothe this effect.
- Apple cider vinegar - 1 tablespoon
- Tea tree essential oil - 5-8 drops

Directions:

1. Mix all the ingredients in a bowl until you have a homogenous mixture.

2. Apply it to your face using your fingertips or a washcloth and gently massage it into the skin for one minute.

3. Rinse off with water, pat dry, and continue with daily activities.

Caution:

Before using apple cider vinegar, you should do a patch test on the inside of your wrist. Rinse off immediately if any irritation occurs because the apple cider vinegar can worsen inflammation. Be careful and avoid contact with the eyes, nose, and mouth. If it happens, rinse thoroughly with water.

Yogurt Cleanser

Yogurt contains lactic acid and probiotics, which makes it perfect for exfoliating the skin while moisturizing and reducing irritation.

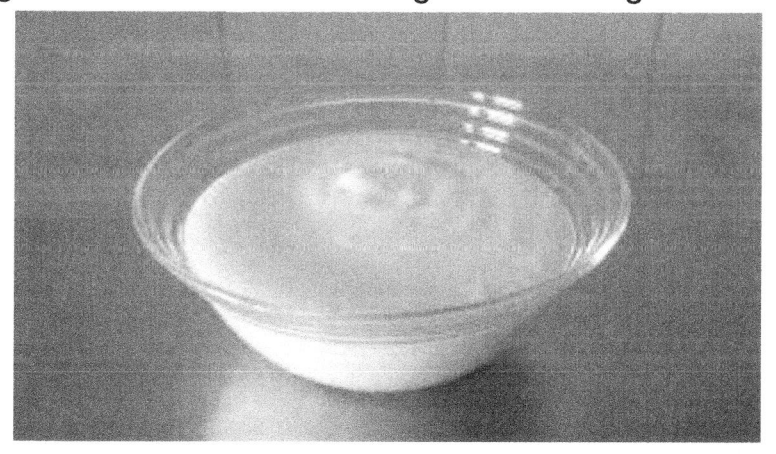

Expert Tip*: If you have extremely sensitive skin, avoid using this cleanser at night because its high-fat content can clog pores if applied while sleeping. It's best to use this cleanser in the morning.*

Ingredients:

- Yogurt- ½ cup (120 ml or 4 oz) - Use full-fat yogurt rich in probiotics, lactic acid, which is excellent for exfoliation and moisturizing the skin without being too harsh.
- Water- ½ cup (120 ml or 4 oz) - Use distilled water if you have hard water or tap water high in impurities, as this can clog pores and create more acne breakouts. This step is optional for those with extremely dry skin types who only want the benefits of yogurt instead of the cleansing effects due to the water content.

Directions:

1. Mix all ingredients in a bowl until you have a smooth paste that is not too runny or thick.

2. Apply it to your face using your fingertips and gently massage it into the skin for one minute before rinsing off with warm water.

3. Pat dry, finish by applying moisturizer – and continue with daily activities.

Toners

Toners are an essential part of the skincare routine. They are used to remove any leftover makeup or dirt after cleansing and are also very important to balance the skin's pH and prepare it for moisturizing (and serums if you choose).

You can make your toner by using fresh ingredients that will be good for your skin. You can also find commercial toners that work well.

Best Toners for Different Skin Types
Different skin types need different toners to get the most out of them.
Dry Skin
You'll want a hydrating, moisturizing toner to help your skin maintain hydration and plump up those fine lines. Look for ingredients like hyaluronic acid (our favorite), glycerin, or shea butter, as they are all moisturizing.
Good Plant-Based Toners for Dry Skin
- **Rosewater Toner** - Rose, glycerin, aloe vera water
- **Aloe Vera Water with Witch Hazel** - Aloe vera extract, witch hazel extract
- **Lavender Chamomile Hydrosol with Balancing Herbs** – Lavender hydrosol, chamomile hydrosol, witch hazel extract
- **Rose Geranium Hydrating Toner** – Rose geranium hydrosol, lavender hydrosol

Sensitive Skin
You'll want a gentle toner that won't irritate your skin. Look for calming ingredients like aloe vera or arnica to soothe and hydrate.
Good Plant-Based Toners for Sensitive Skin
- **Aloe Vera Water with Witch Hazel** – Aloe vera, witch hazel extract
- **Rosewater Toner** – Rosewater, glycerin, aloe vera water
- **Cucumber Hydrating Mist** – Cucumber hydrosol, aloe vera extract
- **Gentle Chamomile Toner** – Lavender hydrosol, chamomile hydrosol

Oily Skin
An astringent toner is best for oily skin. Look for ingredients like witch hazel or apple cider vinegar to help shrink your pores and tighten your skin.
Good Plant-Based Toners for Oily Skin

- **Green Tea Toner** – Green tea extract, witch hazel extract, aloe vera water
- **Apple Cider Vinegar with Rose Water** – Apple cider vinegar, rose water
- **Rose Geranium Hydrating Toner** – Rose geranium hydrosol, lavender hydrosol

Combination Skin

You'll want a toner that can balance both your dry and oily areas. Look for ingredients like aloe vera or witch hazel to keep everything in check.

Good Plant-Based Toners for Combination Skin

- **Rosewater Toner** – Rosewater, glycerin, aloe vera water
- **Lavender Chamomile Hydrosol with Balancing Herbs** – Lavender hydrosol, chamomile hydrosol, witch hazel extract
- **Cucumber Hydrating Mist** – Cucumber hydrosol, aloe vera extract.

How to Use Toner

You can use toner in different ways, depending on your needs.

1. **How to Use Toner as a Cleanser:** You can wipe your face with cotton pads soaked in toner or use a sheet mask for quick cleansing. This way, you won't have to use a separate cleanser each time you cleanse.

2. **How to Use Toner as an Extra Step in your Routine:** This works well for sensitive skin types or if you have oily areas and dry patches (like most of us do!) You can apply it after cleansing but before moisturizing. Then finish up with serums or oils.

DIY Organic Toner Recipes
Rosewater Toner

This is a great all-around toner with rose water, glycerin (a skin-identical ingredient that helps hydration), and aloe vera. You can add witch hazel if you need an astringent for oily areas or chamomile to calm sensitive patches.

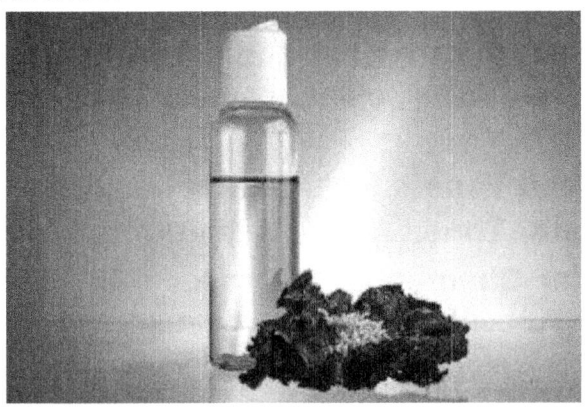

Ingredients:
- Rosewater (30 ml or 1 oz) (store-bought or DIY with roses)
- Glycerin (8-10 drops
- Aloe vera gel (8-10 drops) (options: witch hazel extract, chamomile hydrosol for sensitive skin types)

Expert Tip: *For DIY rosewater, you can use a homemade infusion of roses. Bundle up about 30 buds in cheesecloth and pour boiling water over it to make an infused "tea." You'll want to leave this overnight before using the liquid in your recipe.*

Directions

1. Pour the rosewater into a clean bottle. Add glycerin and aloe vera gel.
2. Shake well to mix them together.
3. You can then add witch hazel extract or chamomile hydrosol if you need it.

Aloe Vera Water with Witch Hazel

This toner is great for dry skin types which need extra hydration. The aloe vera water helps with that, while the witch hazel extract has astringent properties to tighten up your pores after cleansing, which is perfect for oily areas or acne-prone skin.

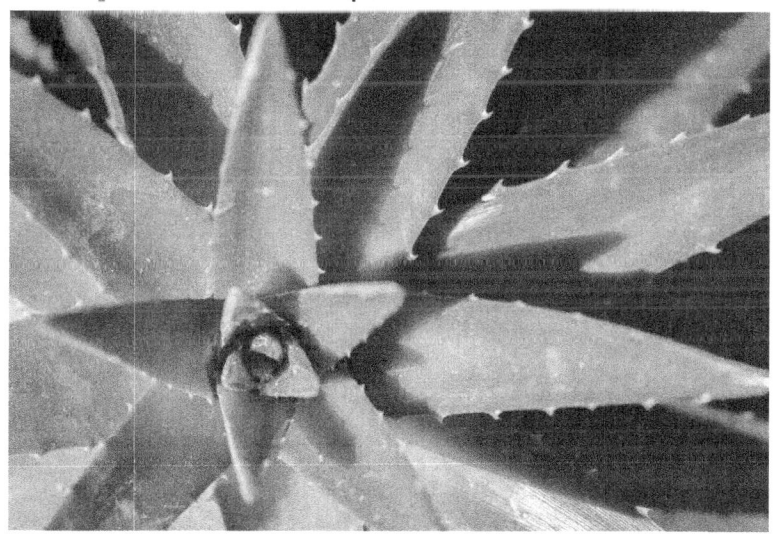

Ingredients:
- Aloe Vera Water (30 ml or about an ounce)
- Witch Hazel Extract (15 drops)

Expert Tip*: For DIY aloe vera water, you can use the gel from an aloe plant. Aloes are easy-to-care-for houseplants with flesh leaves filled with a gooey substance that's great for your skin. To make homemade toner, slice off one of the fat bottom parts of an aloe leaf and squeeze out the gel. Combine that with water in a blender to make it into a liquid, then strain through cheesecloth or any other thin fabric to remove pulp.*

Directions:
1. First, pour the aloe vera water into a clean bottle, followed by witch hazel extract.
2. Shake well before use to mix the two together.

Cucumber Hydrating Mist

This one is also great for dry skin types. It is cooling and refreshing enough to use as an all-over face refresher throughout the day or after workouts on hot days. The cucumber water helps with that, while aloe vera gel soothes and nourishes your skin.

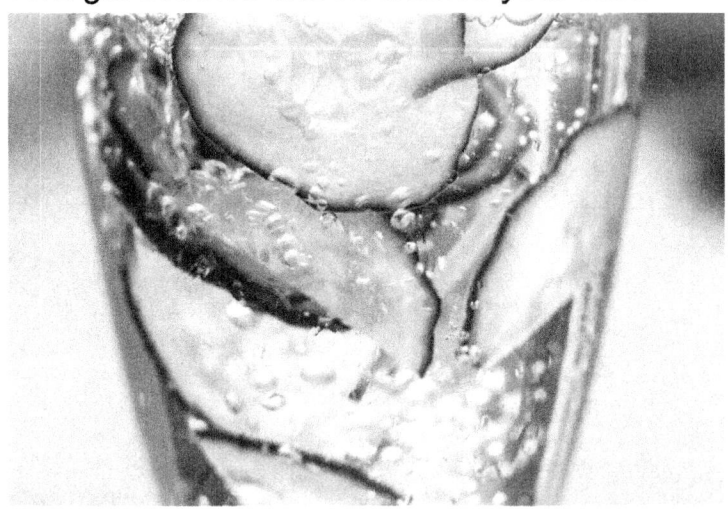

Ingredients:
- Cucumber Hydrosol (30 ml or about an ounce)
- Aloe Vera Gel (15 drops)

Expert Tip*: You can also add a few spritzes of rosewater for extra hydration if you like!*

Directions:

1. Pour the cucumber hydrosol into your clean bottle, followed by aloe vera gel.
2. Shake well to mix them together before use.
3. Store in a cool dark place (like on top of your refrigerator).

Fennel ACV Toner

This toner is great for oily and acne-prone skin types. Fennel helps balance oil production, thanks to its diuretic properties, while apple cider vinegar balances the pH levels of your skin after cleansing, which can reduce breakouts.

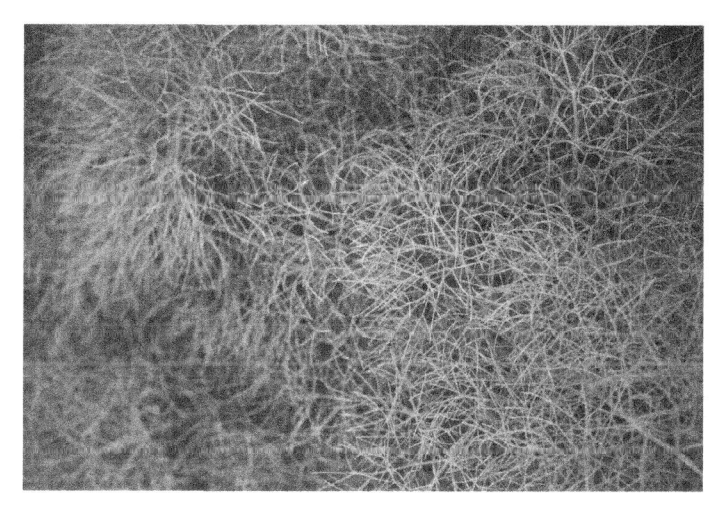

Ingredients:
- Fennel Essential Oil (15 drops)
- Apple Cider Vinegar (15 drops)
- Water or Hydrosol of choice, as needed, to bring the total liquid volume up to 30 ml. or about an ounce.

Expert Tip: *Fennel essential oil can be a little intense for some users with sensitive skin types and may cause irritation with its strong scent. If that's the case, add another essential oil that is soothing and balancing, like lavender or geranium.*

Directions:

1. Combine the fennel essential oil with apple cider vinegar first (you can use water as well if you like).

2. Mix them thoroughly before adding to your bottle of choice, along with any other hydrosols or water, to bring the total liquid volume up to 30 ml.

3. Shake well before use and store in a cool dark place.

Citrus Toner

This toner is great for oily skin types that have clogged pores and/or blackheads and combination skin with dry areas. The lemon essential oil has astringent properties to tighten up your pores after cleansing, while grapefruit hydrosol helps balance the pH levels of your skin and reduces future breakouts.

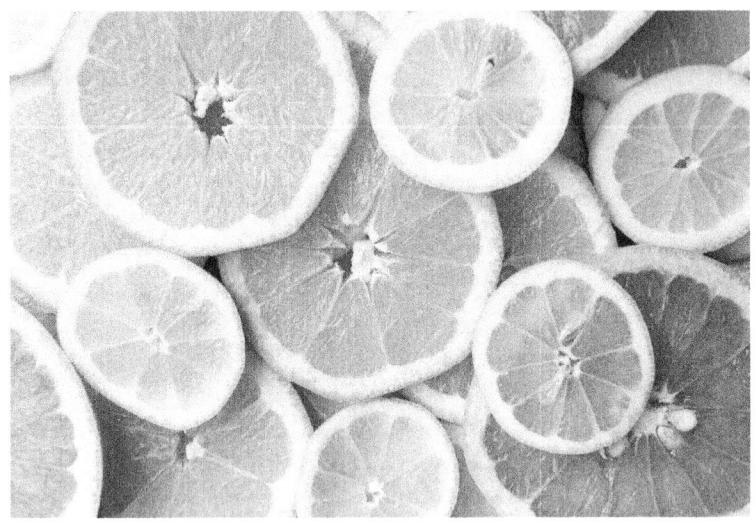

Ingredients:
- Grapefruit Hydrosol (30 ml or about an ounce)
- Lemon Essential Oil (15 drops)

Expert Tip: *You can add a few more drops of lemon essential oil if its scent is too faint for you. Lemons are also great as a dietary supplement to help detox your liver and support healthy cellular function.*

Directions:
1. Combine the grapefruit hydrosol with lemon essential oil first (you can use water as well if you like).
2. Mix them thoroughly before adding to your bottle of choice, along with any other hydrosols or water as needed to bring the total liquid volume up to 30 ml.
3. Shake well before use and store in a cool dark place.

Coconut Rose Toner

This toner is great for dry skin types and sensitive or irritated skin that needs a break after cleansing or exposure to irritating environmental factors like pollutants, smoke, etc. The rose hydrosol helps balance your skin's pH levels, while coconut oil soothes inflammation and nourishes your skin.

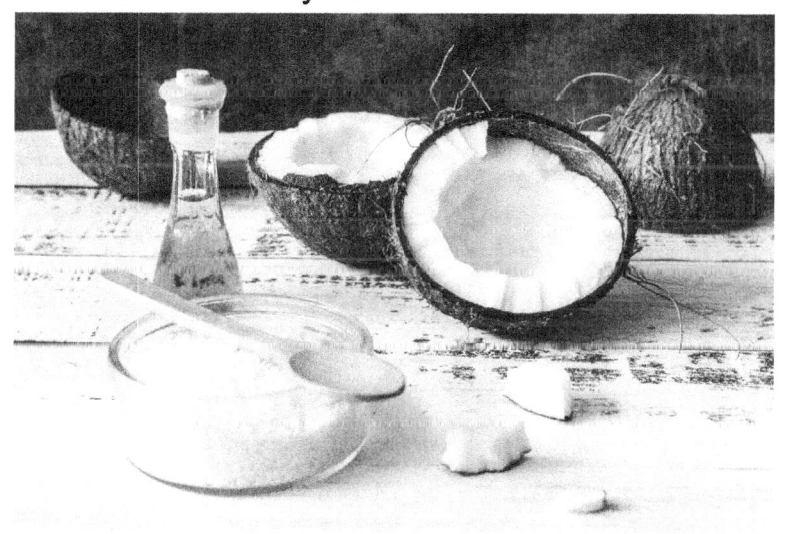

Ingredients:
- Rose Hydrosol (30 ml or about an ounce)
- Coconut Oil (15 drops)

Expert Tip: *You can also add a few spritzes of rosewater for extra hydration if you like! If the coconut oil is too thick for your liking, you can always add some raw honey.*

Directions:

1. Pour the rose hydrosol into a clean bottle first (you can use water as well if you like).

2. Mix them thoroughly before adding to your bottle of choice, along with any other hydrosols or water as needed to bring the total liquid volume up to 30 ml.

3. Gently warm the coconut oil between your fingers before adding it, and add any other essential oils, if desired, for a stronger scent.

4. Shake well before use and store in a cool dark place.

The DIY recipes in this chapter explained how to make organic tinctures for cleansers and toners with ingredients found at your local grocery store or health food market. These easy-to-follow formulas can be customized by adding lavender essential oil for a relaxing fragrance, peppermint oil if you have oily skin, or witch hazel extract if you want an astringent effect on your pores. Now it's time to put these simple steps into action!

Chapter 3: Moisturizers and Face Creams

This chapter will discuss the benefits of moisturizers and face creams. We'll also share some recipes for natural, homemade moisturizers and face creams that you can make at home. These recipes are easy to follow and inexpensive to produce!

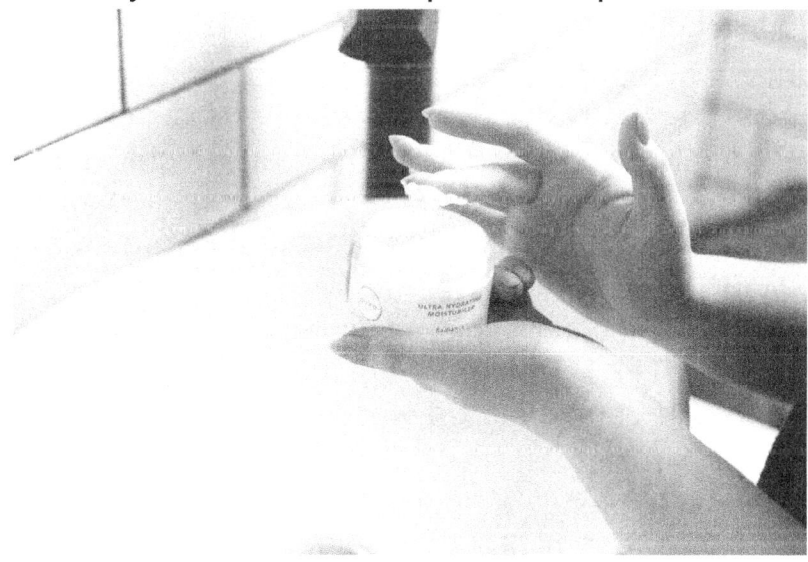

The Difference between a Moisturizer and a Face Cream

A moisturizer is a light, non-greasy cream or lotion that should be used daily to hydrate and nourish your skin. It's essential to use it daily as part of an overall skincare regimen. Moisturizers can contain both natural and synthetic ingredients depending on the brand you select or whether you make it yourself at home with the recipes provided in this book.

A face cream may be more useful for individuals with very dry skin. A good moisturizer won't have any harsh chemicals or additives that can further irritate your skin if it is already highly parched and sensitive due to the cold weather (or air conditioning). If you're looking for something heavier to soothe your dehydrated skin, a face cream would be a better solution.

A moisturizer and a face cream contain ingredients that help hydrate and nourish your skin, but they are not interchangeable as each one serves its purpose depending on where you're using them on your body.

A moisturizer is a blend of ingredients such as water, oil, and emulsifiers that help to hydrate or nourish the skin. In contrast, a face cream is heavier and contains richer ingredients that are great for dry or sensitive skin.

If you have oily and acne-prone skin, a face cream is not ideal as it can cause further breakout problems due to the extra oils present, so you should stick to using moisturizers!

The face cream is used for dryer areas of your body where a moisturizer would not be suitable. It can contain stronger ingredients than those in a moisturizer and will have more beneficial effects on the skin in these cases.

Moisturizers

In a skincare regime, moisturizers are often used after cleansing and toning. Moisturizers hydrate the skin, providing essential nutrients for healthy cell regeneration. They also protect against environmental damage by holding in water to prevent evaporation of moisture from your skin's surface while simultaneously allowing it to breathe naturally.

Moisturizing ingredients include plant oils such as olive, jojoba, castor seed oil, butter such as cocoa butter or shea butter, or beeswax, herbal infusions such as green tea, and calendula.

Moisturizers for Different Skin Types

This section will discuss the different types of moisturizers available and explain how to choose one that best suits your skin type.

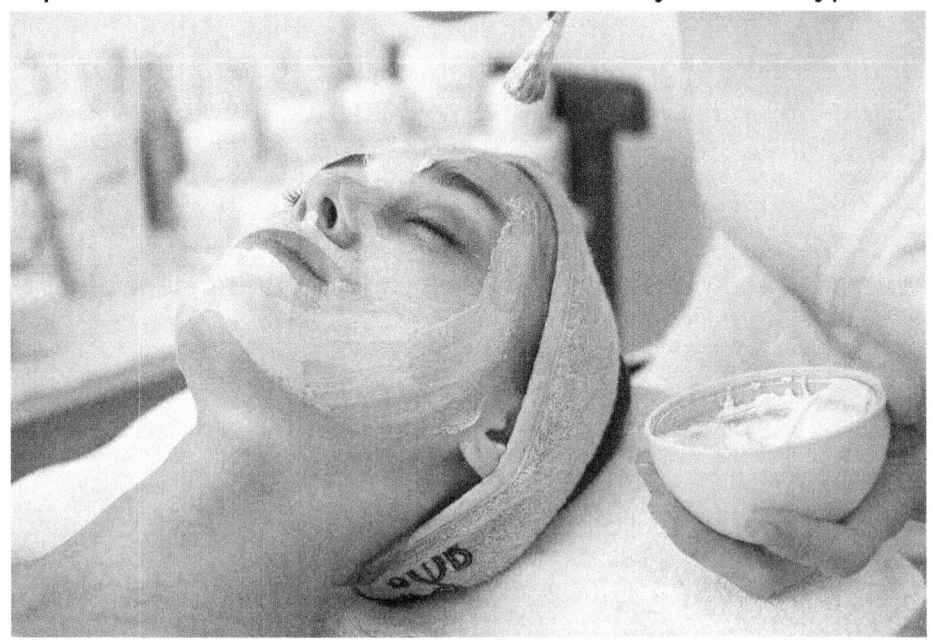

Dry Skin

If you have dry skin, then look for an oil-based moisturizer. Oils are more effective than creams at hydrating the skin because they penetrate deeper and provide moisture to your dermis (the middle layer of your skin).

Oil-based moisturizers should not be used on oily or acne-prone skin as they may clog pores and exacerbate skin problems.

Oily Skin

If you have oily skin, look for a water-based moisturizer as it will not suffocate your skin. Water-based moisturizers effectively hydrate the skin because water is the best natural humectant (attracts and retains moisture). Look for ingredients like hyaluronic acid and glycerin, as they are particularly good at hydrating the skin.

Acne-Prone Skin

If you have acne-prone skin, look for water or oil-based moisturizer that contains ingredients like tea tree leaf extract, known to soothe inflamed and irritated skin while controlling sebum production (the oil your skin naturally produces).

Combination Skin Types

If you have combination skin, look for a moisturizer with ingredients that soothe dryness and hydrate oily areas of the face. Look out for formulations tailored to specific concerns such as dark spots or dull complexion, in addition to normalizing sebum production.

Sensitive Skin

If you have sensitive skin, look for a cream or lotion as they generally do not contain fragrances or dyes. You can also opt for an unscented moisturizer to prevent an adverse reaction.

How to Use a Moisturizer

1. Once you have chosen the best moisturizing ingredients for your skin type, it is time to look at toning and moisturizing the face. The steps are as follows:

2. Cleanse your face with lukewarm water using your fingertips or a washcloth.

3. Apply a toner to remove any leftover dirt on your skin and close the pores with an astringent agent such as witch hazel extract or apple cider vinegar.

4. Moisturize after you have cleansed, exfoliated (optional), and then tone by applying serum and face oil, if desired, using upward strokes.

5. Finish with a sunscreen of SPF 30 or higher to protect your skin from harmful UV rays and prevent signs of aging.

DIY Organic Recipes for Moisturizers

It is very easy to make moisturizers at home. You can use ingredients like aloe vera, honey, green tea extract, and natural oils such as jojoba oil or avocado oil for their anti-inflammatory properties.

Shea Butter Moisturizer for Dry Skin

This moisturizing recipe contains shea butter rich in vitamin A and E. Shea butter also helps protect the skin from UV damage while strengthening skin cells to prevent future damage.

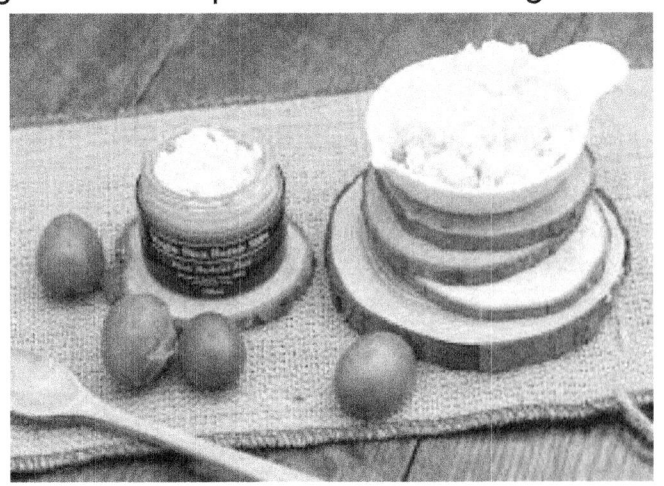

Ingredients:
- ½ tsp of Vitamin E oil (optional)
- ¼ cup raw, organic shea butter
- 15 drops of your favorite essential oils (tea tree, lavender, rosemary)
- ¼ cup organic aloe vera gel (optional)

Directions:

1. Melt shea butter in a double boiler (glass bowl placed over boiling water).

2. If desired, add Vitamin E oil, essential oils, and aloe vera gel. Stir well with a spatula until thoroughly combined.

3. Transfer to a clean glass jar with a metal lid or an old lotion bottle.

Expert Tip: *If you do not have a double boiler, simply place the shea butter in a saucepan and melt on low heat. Stir frequently to prevent burning or sticking.*

Coconut Moisturizer for Oily Skin

This moisturizing recipe contains coconut oil rich in antioxidants and anti-inflammatory properties that help reduce redness in the skin.

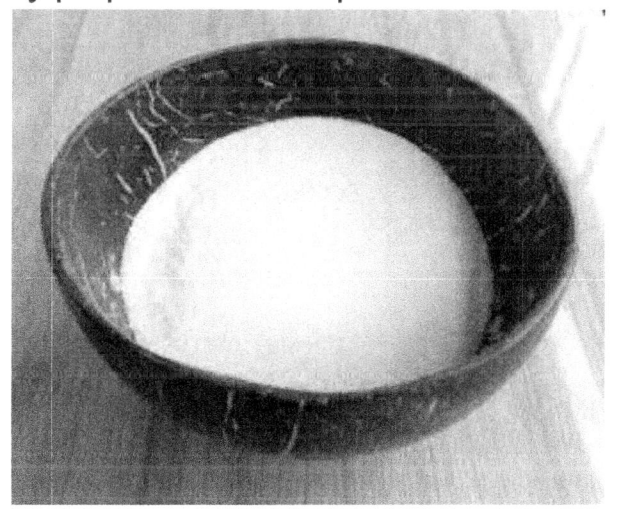

Ingredients:
- ¼ cup raw, organic coconut oil
- 15 drops of your favorite essential oils (eucalyptus, tea tree)
- ¼ cup beeswax pellets

Directions:

1. Melt beeswax in a double boiler (glass bowl placed over boiling water)

2. Remove from heat and add coconut oil and the essential oils. Let the mixture cool to room temperature for about 20 minutes.

3. Transfer to a clean glass jar with a metal lid or an old lotion bottle.

Expert Tip: *Add olive oil and/or glycerin to the recipe for eczema treatment.*

Aloe Vera Moisturizer for Sensitive Skin

This moisturizing lotion contains aloe vera, which is a known soother of inflamed and irritated skin. Aloe vera also helps control sebum production without disrupting the natural balance on your face.

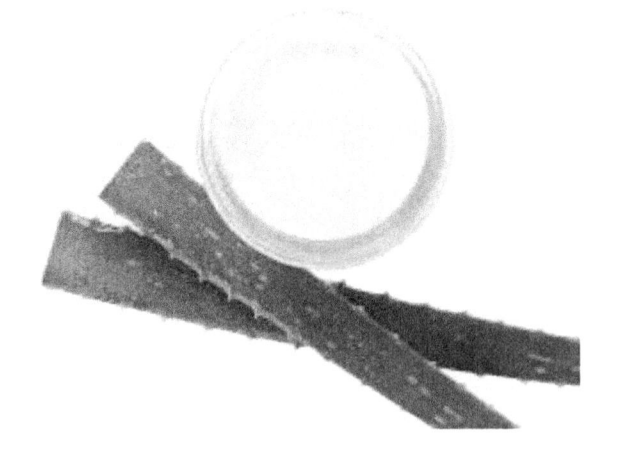

Ingredients:
- ¼ cup raw, organic aloe vera gel
- ½ tsp Vitamin E oil (optional)
- 15 drops of your favorite essential oils (lavender, chamomile, tea tree)

Directions:
1. Add ingredients to a clean glass jar with a metal lid or an old lotion bottle. Shake well to combine.
2. Shake well before each use.

Expert Tip*: Add chamomile and green tea extract to the mixture for a richer moisturizing effect.*

Honey and Glycerin Moisturizer

This moisturizing recipe contains honey and glycerin. Honey helps retain moisture in the skin while providing nourishing antioxidants to reduce redness on your face. Glycerin adds additional hydration to this mixture without leaving any oily residue on the skin, making it perfect for people with oily or acne-prone skin types.

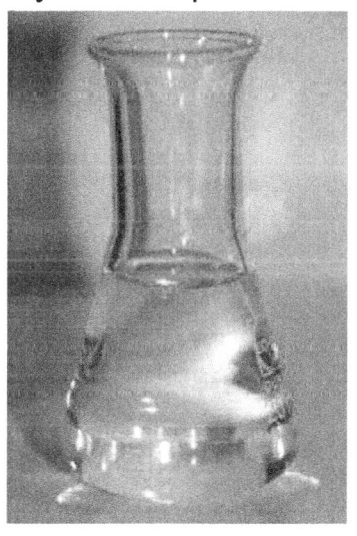

Ingredients:
- ¼ cup raw, organic honey
- ½ tsp glycerin (available at pharmacies and beauty supply stores)
- diluted lemon juice (1 teaspoon)
- green tea (2 teaspoons)

Directions:
1. Combine all ingredients in a glass jar with a metal lid.
2. Shake well to combine before each use.

Expert Tips: *For extra nourishment, add avocado oil and/or coconut milk to the mixture. If you have oily skin, replace honey with organic aloe vera gel.*

Hibiscus Moisturizer for Dry Skin

This moisturizing recipe contains hibiscus tea which is an excellent source of vitamin C and antioxidants. Vitamin C helps stimulate collagen production to improve the appearance of your skin while also reducing signs of aging.

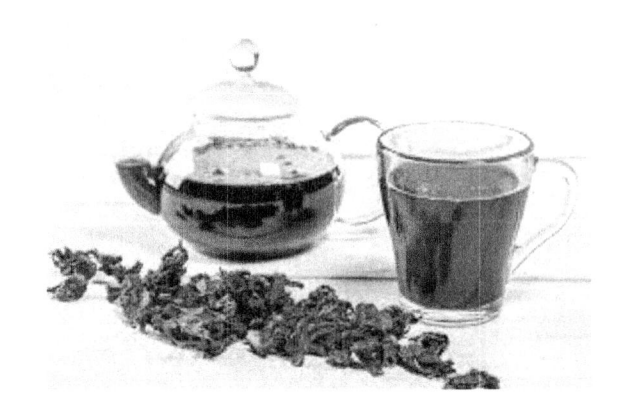

Ingredients:
- 1 cup extra virgin coconut oil
- 2 tablespoons Hibiscus tea in powdered form

Directions:

1. Transfer the coconut oil to a double boiler (a glass bowl placed over boiling water). Melt it on low heat.

2. Add hibiscus tea powder and stir well with a spatula until thoroughly combined. Let it cool for 20 minutes, stirring occasionally.

3. Strain the mixture through a cheesecloth.

4. Whip the mixture with a hand mixer for about one minute.

5. Transfer to an old lotion bottle or clean glass jar with a metal lid.

Expert Tip: *Add green tea extract and/or chamomile extract to the recipe for extra anti-aging benefits. Use Shea butter instead of coconut oil if you have oily skin.*

Face Creams

Different face creams on the market have various benefits, such as lifting and anti-aging properties.

Using a face cream has several benefits, such as:
- Skin becomes more moisturized and hydrated
- It can help minimize fine lines and wrinkles
- Protects skin from the sun's UV rays
- Evens out your skin tone

Face creams are available in different textures, and it feels great on your skin as you apply them.

Face Creams for Different Skin Types

As there are so many different types of face creams available on the market, it can get a bit confusing when choosing the best for your skin type. Always consider your particular skin type when selecting a face cream.

Dry Skin

If you have dry skin, your sebaceous glands do not produce enough oil to keep it moisturized. Therefore, face creams become an essential part of caring for this skin type. Look for a cream with ingredients like Shea butter and glycerin to help hydrate with moisture retention properties.

Oily Skin

If you have oily skin, your sebaceous glands are producing too much oil, which can cause blemishes. Look for a cream with ingredients like salicylic acid and tea tree oil to help prevent pores from becoming clogged and fight acne breakouts.

Combination Skin

Some people's sebaceous glands produce an even amount of oil and moisture, so the skin is neither dry nor oily. Look for a cream with ingredients like glycerin to help keep your face moisturized and witch hazel (which works to give your skin balance.)

Sensitive Skin

If you have sensitive skin, it needs extra care when being treated. Look for a cream with ingredients like aloe vera and chamomile extract to fight irritation caused by dryness, excessive oil production, or blemishes.

Sun-Burnt Skin

If you have sun-burnt skin, then your face may be red and dry. Look for a cream with ingredients like cucumber extract, as this will help soothe the soreness and aloe vera, which is great at moisturizing.

Anti-Aging Creams

There are several different anti-aging creams on the market that work to fight the signs of aging. Look for a cream with ingredients like retinol which will help reduce fine lines and wrinkles, and grape seed extract, which is great at fighting free radicals in your skin.

Lifting Creams

There are creams on the market with lifting properties, and therefore, it's crucial to find one that works for your skin type. Look for a cream with ingredients like firming peptides, which will help to tighten your skin and vitamin C ester to brighten and even out your tone.

How to Use a Face Cream

Using a face cream is very simple. All you need to do is take the desired amount of product on your fingers and gently massage it onto your skin. Let the moisturizer absorb into your skin before applying makeup or any other products.

Organic DIY Recipes for Face Creams

As you may know, organic ingredients are very good for your skin. There are many different recipes out there that use natural ingredients to make face creams at home, such as these:

Shea Butter Face Cream for Smoothening

This homemade face cream is a wonderful way to hydrate and smooth your skin. Jojoba oil and rose water are two very hydrating ingredients to prevent dryness. Shea butter is an excellent moisturizer and anti-inflammatory, so it helps reduce redness and irritation in your skin.

Ingredients:

- 1/3 cup shea butter
- ¼ cup jojoba oil (or other carrier oil)
- 1/8 cup beeswax
- 1/3 cup rose water
- ½ cup aloe gel
- 15 drops essential oil of choice

Directions:

1. In a double boiler, melt beeswax and shea butter until smooth. Remove from heat and allow to cool for about 20 minutes or so (until it's still warm, but you can touch the top without burning your fingers).

2. Add carrier oil of choice, if needed. Jojoba works best in this recipe because it's very light and gets absorbed easily into the skin. However, you can substitute another carrier oil of your choice.

3. Add aloe gel and essential oils of your choice. Blend on high until smooth and creamy.

4. Pour into a jar or container and let it cool completely before putting on the lid. If stored properly in a cool, dry place away from direct sunlight, you can keep it for up to six months.

Expert Tip: *If you don't have a double boiler to melt your ingredients, you can place a glass or metal bowl over a saucepan with about an inch of water in it. Make sure the bottom of the bowl does not touch the simmering water.*

Rosemary Honey Face Cream for Acne-Prone Skin

This face cream is wonderful for those who suffer from acne and oily skin. The rosemary and honey work together to help cleanse your pores and fight any bacteria that may be causing the breakouts.

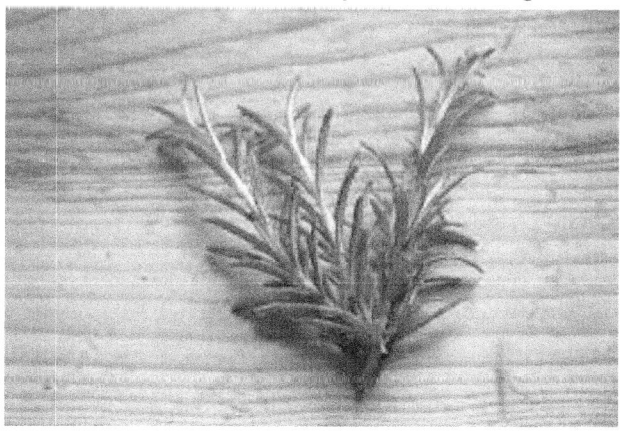

Ingredients:

- ½ cup raw Honey
- ¼ cup Coconut Oil (melted)
- ½ tsp Fresh or Dried Rosemary Leaves, finely chopped
- ¼ cup Beeswax

Directions:

1. Using a double boiler, melt the coconut oil and beeswax until smooth. Remove from heat.

2. Add honey and rosemary leaves to melted ingredients in the pan. Stir well to combine.

3. Pour the mixture into a container of your choice. Let it cool completely before putting it on the lid. If stored properly in a cool, dry place away from direct sunlight, you can keep it for up to six months.

Expert Tip: *If you don't want to use coconut oil, you can substitute it with any other carrier oil of your choice.*

Anti-Wrinkle Face Cream

This face cream is perfect for those who have wrinkles and dry skin. The avocado in this recipe works well to moisturize your skin while providing a natural source of antioxidants that will help protect the collagen from free radicals, which can cause signs of aging.

Ingredients:

- 15 grams/0.53 oz Avocado Oil
- 10 grams/0.35 oz Argan Oil
- 15 grams/0.53 oz Emulsifying Wax NF
- 300 grams/10.58 oz Boiled water (or ready-made hydrosol)
- 1 handful Dried Calendula Flowers (not required if using ready-made hydrosol)
- 1 grams/0.04 oz Preservative (optional)
- 15 drops Frankincense Essential Oil
- 10 drops Lemon Essential Oil

Directions:

1. Make a herbal mixture with 10 fl oz (300 grams) of boiling water and a handful of Calendula flowers. To make an herbal infusion, put the flowers into a jar, pour boiling water on top, then cover it to cool.

2. If you don't want to make the infusion, you may use a ready-made floral hydrosol.

3. Melt the oils (make sure not to boil them). Once melted, combine the water and oils. Mix well gently with a spoon or a whisk without forming any bubbles. Once the mixture starts to emulsify, you may add the preservative if you wish to. Add the oils once the mixture reaches room temperature.

Expert Tip: *If you don't add a preservative, the cream should be kept in the fridge and used up within a few days.*

Face Cream for Sunburns

This face cream is great for those who have sunburn. The aloe vera and raw honey work together to help heal your skin while providing a light moisturizing effect that won't leave you feeling greasy or sticky

Ingredients:
- 1/3 cup Aloe Vera Gel
- 1/3 cup Shea Butter
- 1/3 cup Raw Honey

Directions:

1. In a double boiler, melt the shea butter and aloe vera gel until smooth and creamy (if you don't have a double boiler, you can melt them in a glass or metal bowl placed over a saucepan with about an inch of water).

2. Once the mixture is smooth and creamy, remove it from heat. Add honey, and stir well to combine. Pour into a container of your choice, let it cool completely before putting on the lid.

3. Apply this cream overnight, and in the morning, rinse it off with lukewarm water and pat dry.

Expert Tip: *If you don't like using Shea Butter, feel free to use another type of butter such as cacao or mango butter (or even coconut oil) instead.*

Eye Creams

This eye cream is great for dark circles and/or fine lines around their eyes. The coconut oil, avocado oil, and vitamin E work together to help hydrate your skin and protect it from escalating the signs of aging.

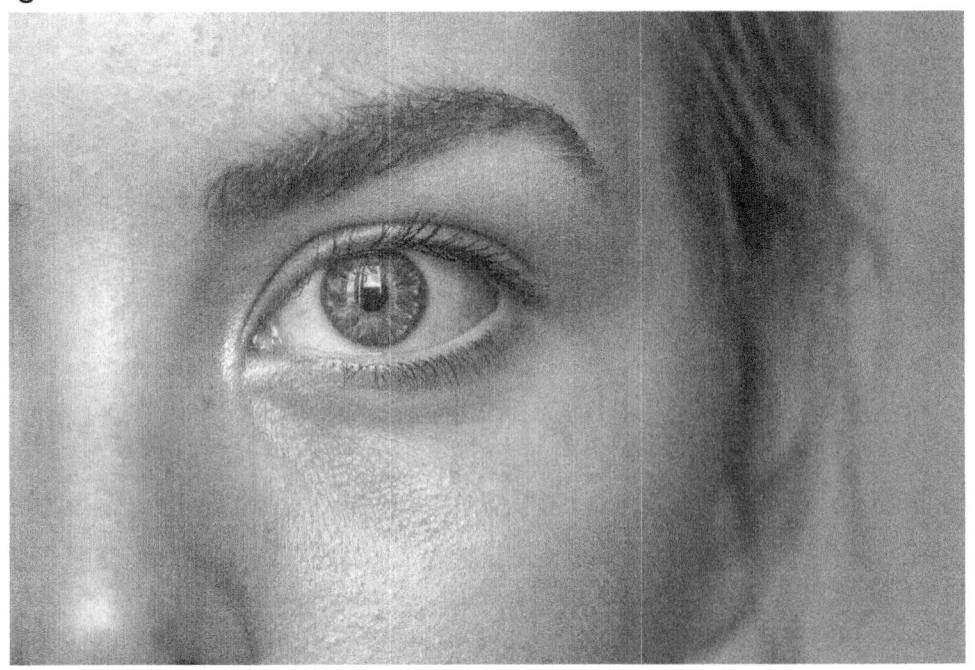

Ingredients:
- Vitamin-E Capsules (make sure they are pure and without any additives)
- Coconut Oil
- ½ teaspoon Avocado oil or Sweet Almond oil. If you don't like the smell of avocado oil, feel free to use another type of carrier oil such as olive oil, jojoba seed, etc.

Directions:
1. Cut open a vitamin E capsule and pour the contents into a clean, empty bowl.

2. Add coconut oil and whip until creamy with a hand mixer or stand mixer (if you don't have one, feel free to use your hands instead).

3. If necessary, add more capsules of Vitamin E and carrier oils of your choice. Whip until the mixture is fluffy and creamy, then transfer it into a glass jar with a lid for storage.

The recipes in this chapter should help you create your DIY facial moisturizers and face creams without buying expensive ingredients or equipment. The best thing about these products is that they are customizable based on what works for your skin type, how dry it is, the temperature of your environment, etc. If one recipe doesn't work out well for you, try another!

Remember: there's no such thing as a perfect formula, so experiment with different ingredients until you find something that meets your needs perfectly.

Chapter 4: Natural Scrubs for Your Face and Body

The fourth chapter in this series is about natural scrubs that can be used on your face and body. We will go over how to make the scrub, what they are most useful for, and why they work so well.

What Is a Scrub?

A scrub is a product that helps to exfoliate the skin.

Exfoliation means removing dead or dying cells from the surface of your body, leaving healthy and glowing skin underneath. Scrubs are most commonly made with salt, sugar, cocoa seeds (cocoa powder), coffee grounds/beans, or nutshells as the exfoliating ingredient.

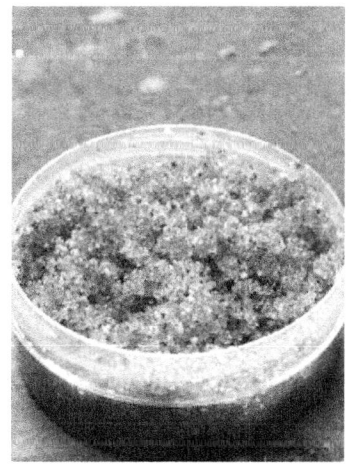

Scrubs can be used on your face and body to help remove dead skin cells, promote healthy blood flow, improve the appearance of cellulite by reducing fluid retention in fatty tissue under the skin, and prevent and diminish stretch marks and scars.

A scrub is a powdered mixture containing tiny little beads, which help exfoliate the skin. Scrubs are used in many different stages of skincare and beauty treatments, such as facials or body wraps.

Benefits of Using a Scrub in Your Skin Care Regime

There are many benefits of using a scrub in your skin care regime. Some of the most common benefits include:

- Reduces the appearance of cellulite by reducing fluid retention and promoting healthy blood flow.
- Exfoliation leaves skin feeling smooth, refreshed, and rejuvenated.
- Removes dead skin cells, which can help improve skin tone and texture.
- It helps to reduce the appearance of acne scars, stretch marks, and other imperfections.

These are just a few benefits you can expect from using a scrub in your skin care regime. It is important to remember that scrubs should not be used on broken or irritated skin as they can cause further irritation and damage.

Face Scrub vs. Body Scrub

The most typical difference between facial scrubs and body scrubs is the ingredients.

Facial scrub ingredients typically include natural oils, water, sugar, or sea salt as exfoliating agents, with added essential oils for fragrance. Face scrub recipes are generally gentler on your skin since they are designed to be used in a smaller area where you have more delicate skin.

Most body scrubs typically use sugar or salt as the exfoliating agent and do not contain a lot of fragrances, essential oils, or added moisturizers as you would find in a facial scrub recipe. Body scrub recipes are generally more efficient at removing dead skin cells, which is why they work so well on other areas of your body, such as your arms and legs.

It is important to note that a body scrub should not be used on your face as it can cause irritation and damage to the skin. This is because body scrub ingredients are usually harsher than those found in facial scrubs.

Facial Scrubs

Facial scrubs can be used on your face and neck area to remove dead skin cells, improve blood flow to help promote healthy cell growth in new skin tissue, improve the appearance of cellulite, and reduce stretch marks.

There are different ways to make a facial scrub, depending on what you want it to do for your skin. You can use raw cane sugar or sea salt as both are exfoliants, in addition to natural oils such as coconut oil or olive oil, which help to moisturize and nourish your skin.

You can also add in the benefits of essential oils by adding a few drops to your facial scrub before you mix it. Essential oils are known for their skin-friendly properties and work great as natural fragrances!

How to Use a Facial Scrub

To use a facial scrub, all you have to do is gently massage the mixture onto your face and neck area for about two minutes.

After giving it a gentle rub for at least two minutes, rinse the scrub off with cold water and pat dry with a clean towel.

Frequency

It is recommended to use a facial scrub about twice per week, but you can increase or decrease the frequency depending on your skin type and needs.

Types of Facial Scrubs for Different Skin Types

Depending on your skin type, you may need to use a different facial scrub recipe from that used by someone else.

Suppose you have dry, sensitive, or mature skin. In that case, it is best to stick with sugar scrubs because they are generally less harsh on the skin and can help reduce the appearance of fine lines and wrinkles over time. If you're looking for something a little gentler, then you can try a scrub with almond or jojoba oil as the exfoliant. This is also good for dry skin because these oils moisturize and nourish the skin without causing irritation.

If you have oily, acne-prone, or combination skin types, it would be best to stick with a facial scrub that uses salt as the exfoliant. Salt is a much more effective exfoliator than sugar and works well for oily skin because it helps absorb excess oil without causing breakouts or irritation.

If you are looking to minimize the appearance of fine lines, wrinkles, or hyperpigmentation, then it would be best to try a facial scrub with essential oils as the exfoliant. Essential oils are known for their anti-aging properties and work great in improving blood flow which can help reduce the appearance of stretch marks, scars from acne breakouts, or hyperpigmentation caused by hormonal imbalance or sun damage.

DIY Organic Recipes for Facial Scrubs

We have gathered a few of our favorite DIY recipes for facial scrubs that you can try out:

Brown Sugar Face Scrub (for Dry and Mature Skin)

This recipe is best for those with dry, sensitive, and mature skin.

Ingredients:
- ¼ cup Brown Sugar (can also use raw cane sugar)
- ½ tablespoon Jojoba Oil or Almond Oil
- A few drops of Rose Essential Oil (optional, but recommended for dry and/or aging skin types)

Directions:
1. Mix all ingredients in a small bowl and rub onto your face in a circular motion for two minutes.
2. Rinse off with cold water to reveal your fresh, moisturized skin!

Sugar and Sea Salt Scrub (for Oily Skin)

This recipe is best for those who have oily, acne-prone skin types.

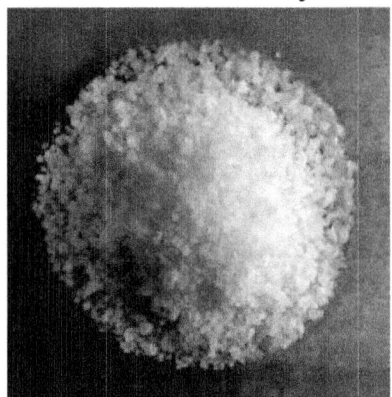

Ingredients:
- ¼ cup Sea Salt
- ½ tablespoon Coconut Oil

Directions:

1. Mix all ingredients in a small bowl and rub onto your face in a circular motion for two minutes.

2. Rinse off with cold water to reveal your fresh, moisturized skin!

Strawberry Face Scrub (for All Skin Types)

This recipe is best for those with dry, sensitive skin. Strawberries are known to be a little gentler on the skin than other fruits and work great as an exfoliant.

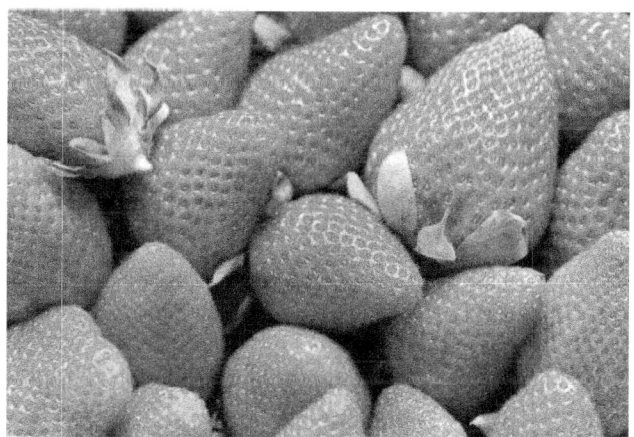

Ingredients:
- ¼ cup Strawberries (fresh or frozen)
- ½ tablespoon Jojoba Oil (or almond oil)

Directions:

1. Mix all ingredients in a blender until you get your desired consistency.

2. Rub onto your face in a circular motion for two minutes and rinse off with cold water to reveal your fresh, clean skin!

Lemon Face Scrub (for Sensitive Skin)

This recipe is best for those who have dry or mature skin types. Lemons are known as natural astringents that can help tighten up pores and minimize the appearance of fine lines and wrinkles.

Ingredients:

- ½ Lemon (fresh or frozen)
- ¼th cup Brown Sugar (can also use raw cane sugar)

Directions:

Mix all ingredients in a small bowl and rub onto your face in a circular motion for two minutes. Rinse off with cold water to reveal your fresh, cleansed skin!

Coffee Scrub (for All Skin Types)

This recipe is best for those with oily or combination skin types because coffee grounds are great at absorbing excess oil.

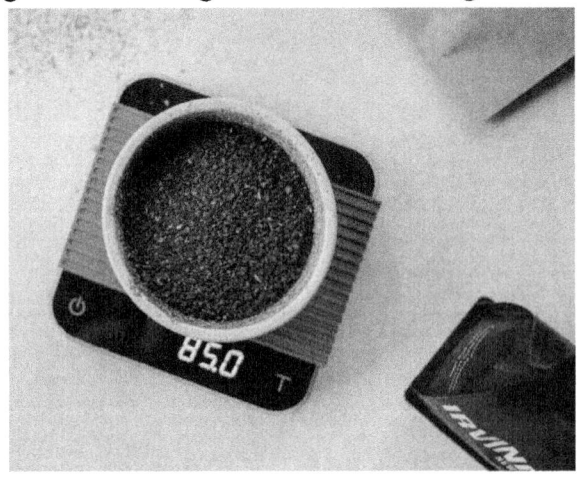

Ingredients:

- ¼ cup Coffee Grounds (or you can use a teaspoon of instant or espresso powder)
- ½ tablespoon Jojoba Oil (can also use almond, coconut, or olive oil)

Directions:

1. Mix all ingredients in a small bowl and rub onto your face in a circular motion for two minutes.
2. Rinse off with cold water to reveal your fresh, clean skin!

Oatmeal Scrub (for All Skin Types)

This recipe is best for those who have dry, sensitive skin types. Oatmeal contains beta-glucan, which has been known to help calm

down inflammation and itchiness on the skin.
Ingredients:
- ½ tablespoon Oatmeal (either ground or in flakes - you can use a blender if needed)
- ¼ cup Brown Sugar (can also use raw cane sugar)

Directions:
1. Mix all ingredients in a small bowl and rub onto your face in a circular motion for two minutes.
2. Rinse off with cold water to reveal your fresh, clean skin!

Aloe Vera Scrub (for Dry Skin)

This recipe is best for those who have dry or mature skin types. Aloe vera is known for its moisturizing and soothing properties, which work great at hydrating the skin and preventing fine lines, wrinkles, sunspots, and dark circles under the eyes.

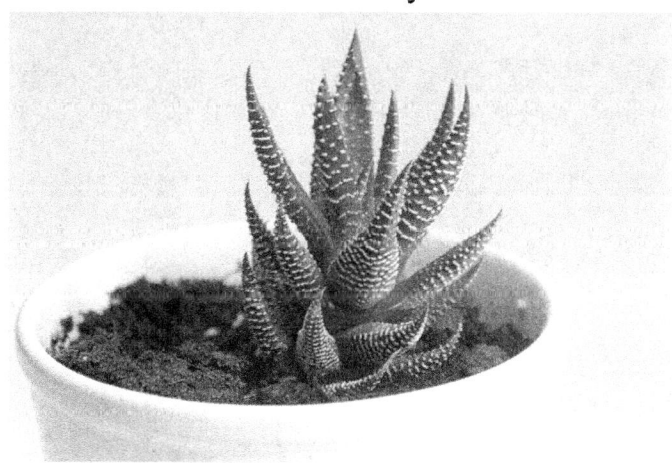

Ingredients:
- A few drops of Aloe Vera Gel (can also use rosehip seed oil)
- ¼ cup raw Cane Sugar (can also use brown or coconut sugar)

Directions:

1. Mix all ingredients in a small bowl and rub onto your face in a circular motion for two minutes.

2. Rinse off with cold water to reveal your fresh, moisturized skin!

Citrus Sugar Scrub (for All Skin Types)

This recipe is best for those with oily or combination skin types because the citric acid in oranges helps cut through excess oil. Oranges are also known as great astringents that can help tighten pores and reduce the appearance of blackheads.

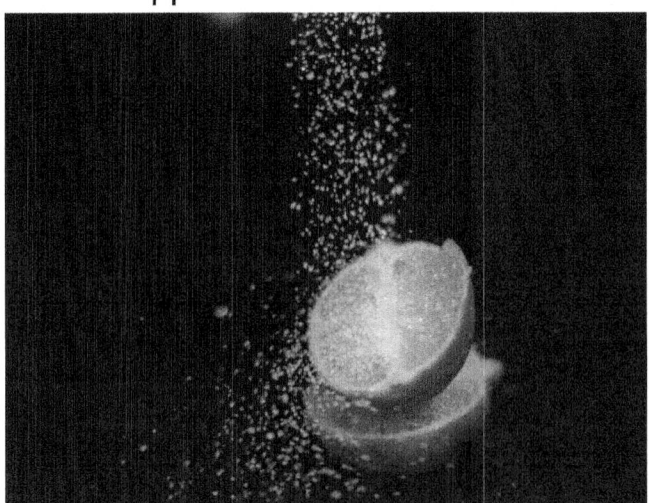

Ingredients:
- ½ orange (fresh or frozen)
- ¼ cup raw Cane Sugar (can also use brown or coconut sugar)

Directions:

1. Mix all ingredients in a small bowl and rub onto your face in a circular motion for two minutes.

2. Rinse off with cold water for clean and refreshed skin.

Neem Oil Scrub (for All Skin Types)

This recipe is best for those who have oily or combination skin types because neem oil is great at balancing out the pH levels of the skin and reducing excess sebum (oil) production.

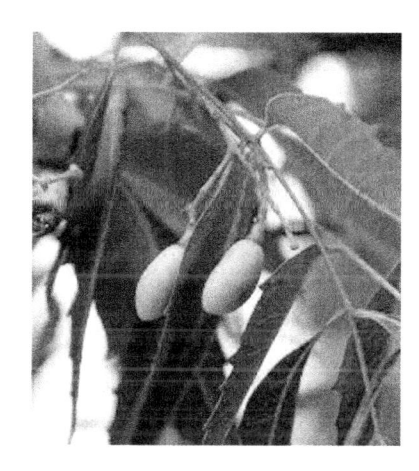

Ingredients:
- ¼ cup raw Cane Sugar (can also use brown, coconut sugar)
- ½ tablespoon Neem Oil (you can substitute this for coconut oil)

Directions:

1. Mix all ingredients in a small bowl and rub onto your face in a circular motion for two minutes. Rinse off with cold water to reveal your fresh, clean skin!

2. You may use any combination of these recipes to create your own natural scrub. All you have to do is mix the dry ingredients with a carrier oil (jojoba, coconut, or olive) and store them in an airtight container!

Body Scrubs

A body scrub is a great way to exfoliate the skin and get rid of dead, flaky skin cells. Exfoliation helps to improve circulation in the area, which will help with collagen production.

How to Use a Body Scrub
- Make sure to cleanse the skin first
- Apply the scrub all over the body using small, circular motions so that you don't have too much of the product on any one area of your skin.
- Let it sit for a few minutes before rinsing off with warm water to reveal soft and smooth skin!

Body Scrubs for Different Skin Types

Remember to use the right ingredients to get rid of dead skin cells, fight acne, and improve your skin's overall health. Here are a few recipes depending on what skin type you have!

- For those with **oily or combination skin types**, try out a coffee body scrub because it will help decrease the amount of sebum production on your face while tightening pores at the same time.
- For those with **dry skin,** try out a coconut oil body scrub! Coconut oil is known for its moisturizing properties and will keep your skin hydrated throughout the day. It also contains fatty acids, which help improve collagen production - that's why it's great to combat fine lines and wrinkles.
- For those of you with a **normal skin type,** try out a pear body scrub. Pears are full of antioxidants that help improve your complexion, fight off dark spots from sun damage and prevent signs of aging such as fine lines, deep-set wrinkles, and sagging skin. They also stimulate collagen production, so you'll have more elastic skin, which will help prevent stretch marks!
- For those with **sensitive skin types,** try out a coffee body scrub because it contains caffeine which helps get rid of dark circles. It also tightens pores and reduces acne breakouts to have clear, blemish-free skin. Coffee is full of antioxidants that fight off premature aging signs, while sugar helps exfoliate your skin.
- For those with **combination or oily skin types,** try out a cocoa powder body scrub! Cocoa powder contains antioxidants that help reduce the appearance of dark spots, which is excellent in evening out your complexion and preventing acne breakouts. At the same time, coconut oil acts as an anti-inflammatory to prevent redness.

DIY Organic Body Scrub Recipes

Here are a few body scrub recipes you can try out at home. Remember, always use organic ingredients! Making a scrub is super easy - all you have to do is mix the dry ingredients with a carrier oil (jojoba, coconut, or olive) and store them in an airtight container. It is also easy to create a fresh batch each time you use it.

Coconut Oil and Cocoa Powder Body Scrub

This is great for those with normal to dry skin because the cocoa powder will help lock in moisture, and coconut oil is known for its antioxidant properties.

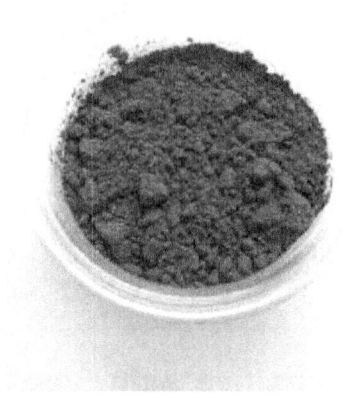

Ingredients:
- Coconut Oil (as needed)
- Cocoa Powder (as needed)

Directions:
1. Mix ingredients and use them as a body scrub.
2. Depending on how moisturizing you want the scrub to be, you can add more or less.

Pear and Blueberry Body Scrub

This is great for those with normal skin because pears are full of antioxidants that help fight fine lines, improve complexion, and promote cellular health, while blueberries contain powerful antioxidants that can help prevent dark spots from sun damage!

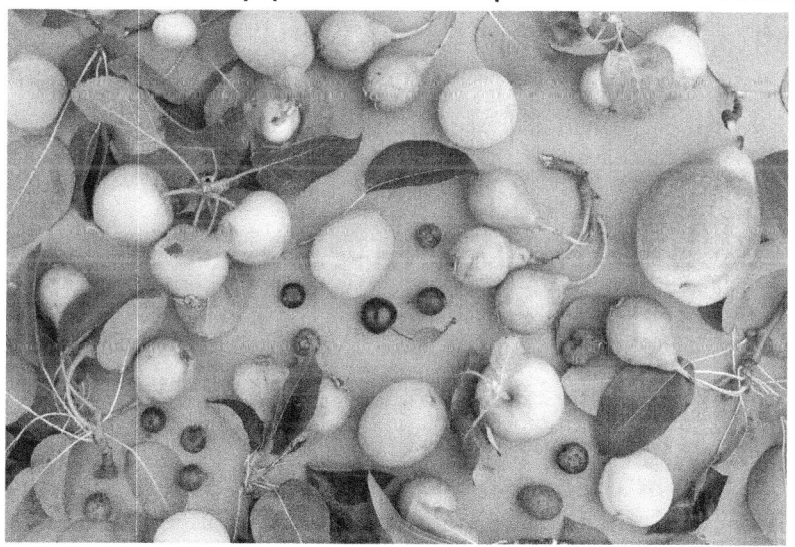

Ingredients:
- Blueberries (as needed)
- Pear (as needed)

Directions:
1. Cleanse your skin, and then mash together the blueberries with the pear.
2. Apply all over your body in small, circular motions.
3. Rinse off after two minutes to reveal soft skin! You can also add raw cane sugar if you want more of a scrub.

Coffee Body Scrub

This is great for those with normal skin because the caffeine in coffee helps stimulate circulation, which, in turn, helps to tighten the pores, reduce dark circles, and improve under-eye bags! The raw cane sugar also acts as an exfoliant to remove dead skin cells while the coconut oil hydrates it.

Ingredients:
- Ground Coffee (as needed)

- Coconut Oil (as needed)
- Raw Cane Sugar

Directions:

1. Take a small amount of ground coffee and mix with coconut oil until it becomes a paste.

2. Add in the raw cane sugar as you would to your regular body scrub recipe.

3. Apply all over your body, let sit for two minutes.

4. Rinse off with warm water for clean skin that's free from impurities.

Clay and Almond Milk Body Scrub

This is great for those with normal skin because the clay and almond milk act as a natural detoxifier which will help improve complexion, shrink pores, and tighten your skin!

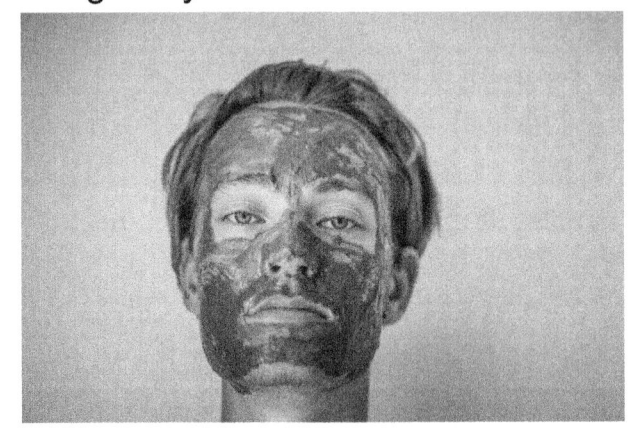

Ingredients:

- Clay (1/2 Cup)
- Almond Milk (1/2 Cup)
- Honey (as needed)

Directions:

1. Mix all ingredients until it becomes a paste.

2. Apply over your skin and rinse off after five minutes.

3. Depending on how moisturizing you want the scrub to be, you can use more or less clay. Remember, always do a patch test before using new ingredients on your face or body.

Coconut Oatmeal Sugar Body Scrub

This is great for those with normal to dry skin because coconut oil and oatmeal will help hydrate your skin while exfoliating it at the same time! Raw cane sugar acts as an anti-inflammatory which helps in reducing redness and preventing acne breakouts.

Ingredients:
- Coconut Oil (2-3 tablespoons)
- Oatmeal (1/4 cup)
- Raw Cane Sugar (1/2 cup)

Directions:

1. Melt coconut oil in the microwave for about 30 seconds to a minute.

2. Combine raw cane sugar and oatmeal in a small bowl, then add melted coconut oil into the mixture until it becomes a paste.

3. You should not need any water to create this scrub. After cleansing, apply the product all over your body, and let it sit for three minutes.

4. Rinse off with warm water for clean skin that's free from impurities.

Matcha Green Tea Body Scrub

This is great for those with normal to dry skin because matcha green tea will help protect your body from free radical damage, which can cause fine lines, wrinkles, and sagging! Matcha is an excellent antioxidant and helps control redness and acne breakouts.

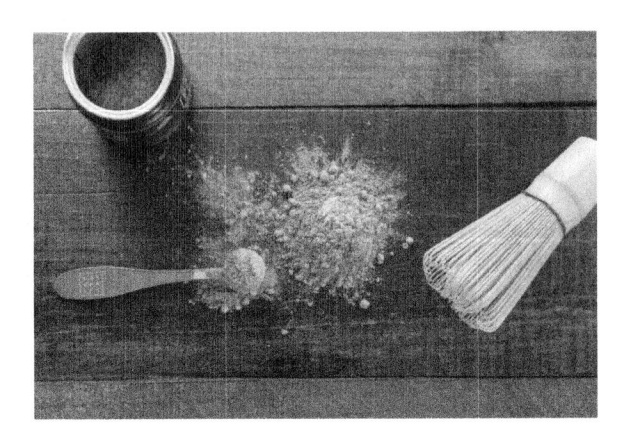

Ingredients:
- Matcha Green Tea Powder (1 teaspoon)
- 1 Cup Sugar
- Plain Green Tea (1 teaspoon)
- Jojoba Oil as a carrier

Directions:

1. Mix the matcha green tea powder with one cup of sugar, then add in some plain green tea and jojoba oil.
2. Mix well until it becomes a paste, and apply all over your body.
3. Let it sit for two to three minutes, depending on how moisturizing you want the scrub to be.
4. Rinse off with warm water.

Rosehip Oil Body Scrub

Rosehip oil is great for those with dry skin because it contains essential fatty acids that help improve your complexion, reduce fine lines, and smooth out the surface of your skin. It is also rich in vitamins A and E, which help reduce skin aging.

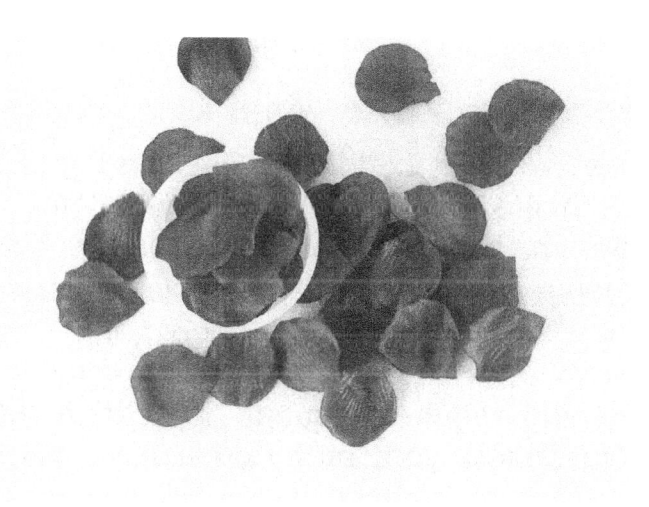

Ingredients:
- 1 cup fine Sugar
- 1/4 Cup Olive Oil
- 1 tablespoon Rosehip Oil

Directions:
1. Mix all ingredients until it becomes a paste.
2. Apply over the skin and rinse off after five minutes.

In this concluding paragraph, we want to reiterate that a good scrub is an instant way to rejuvenate your skin without having to go under the knife or spend hours at a spa. There are many benefits associated with using a facial scrub regularly, including reduced inflammation, decreased acne breakouts, reduced oiliness or dryness as well as having improved circulation. You can use these recipes in conjunction or independently, depending on what your specific needs happen to be. Keep reading if you're interested in learning how easy it is to make serums and face masks!

Chapter 5: Serums and Masks

In this chapter, we will explore serums and masks. Serums and masks are both great ways to hydrate your skin, but what's the difference? Serums typically contain a higher concentration of active ingredients than a face mask does. This is because serums usually include ingredients that penetrate deeper into the skin, such as retinol or vitamin C. The downside to using serums is that they can be expensive and require frequent application. Masks provide a temporary solution for hydration by providing a barrier on the skin's surface from external irritants, which allows for deep penetration from other topical products.

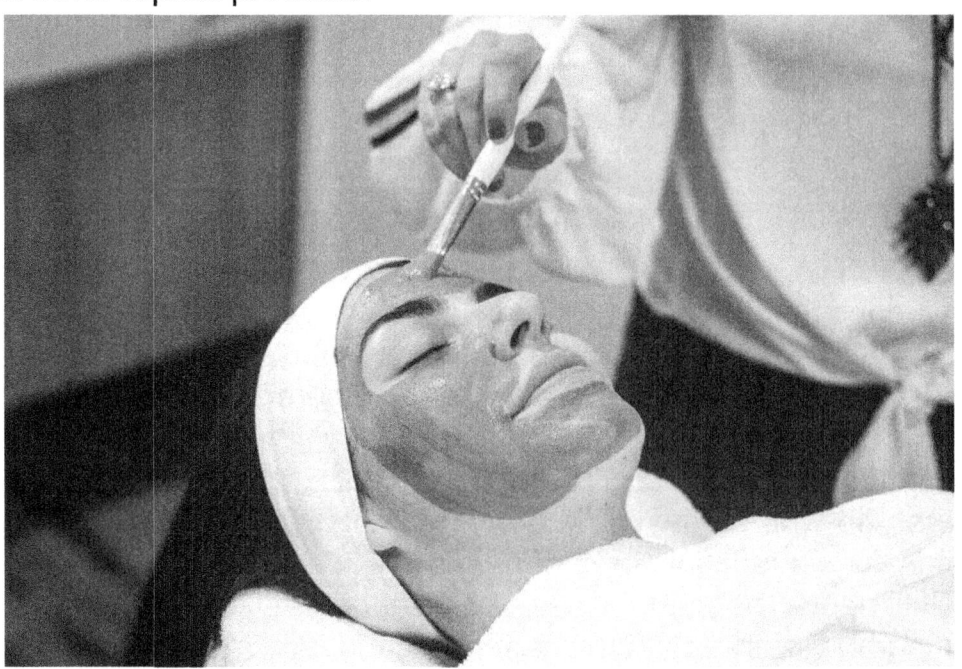

Difference between a Mask and a Serum

There is a big difference between serums and masks. Serums are typically thinner in consistency, as they have to penetrate deeper into the skin for optimal benefits. The reason why masks tend to be thicker is that there needs to be enough of the product on your face so that it can dry out before you rinse it away.

The other key difference is that masks are applied for a longer duration than serums, which typically last around 20 minutes or so before they are rinsed off. This happens because some types of masks need sufficient time for their ingredients to bond with your skin.

Masks tend to be a bit more focused on the skin's surface, whereas serums penetrate deeper into the skin and provide benefits below the surface of your pores.

In addition, serums typically moisturize better than facial masks.

Face Serums

Face Serums are one of the most important products in any skin care regimen. They are used to deliver special ingredients deep into your skin, where they can work their magic on a cellular level.

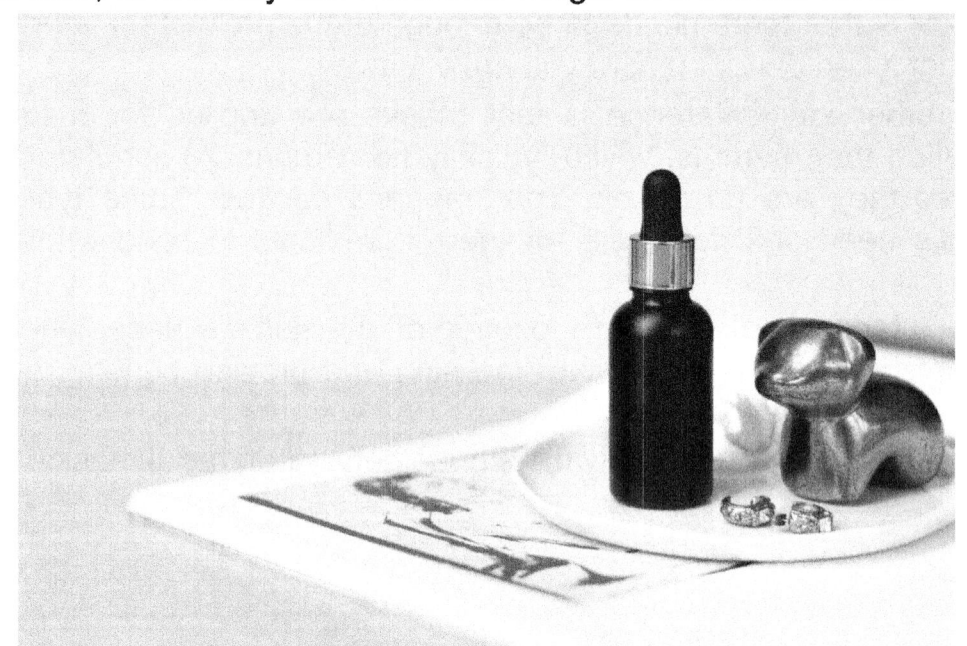

There are many face serums available for different skin types and concerns. Some contain hyaluronic acid or collagen to plump up fine lines, while others are loaded with vitamins A, C, or E to protect the skin from environmental aggressors.

Serums will give you maximum results in minimal time. They can be used on their own, but many women find them too rich for day use and prefer to reserve them for night-time routine only. It is important to avoid using heavy moisturizers under your serum as this can cause them to pill up or slip off the skin altogether.

Serums are perfect for all skin types, including sensitive and acne-prone ones. They tend to be more expensive than face creams, but a little goes a long way with these powerhouse products!

Serums for Different Skin Issues

Serums serve many purposes but are especially effective for addressing specific skin issues.

Anti-Aging

Hyaluronic acid is one of the most popular ingredients in anti-aging serums. Hyaluronic acid acts like a sponge, soaking up water and helping to plump out fine lines while also adding much-needed hydration back into dry skin. Look for these types of serum if you're looking to fight the signs of aging.

Brightening/Hyperpigmentation

Evening out your skin tone and texture is a great way to diminish hyperpigmentation or dark spots. Vitamin C serums are ideal for brightening up dull, lackluster complexions. They promote cell turnover on a deeper level than typical face moisturizers.

Acne/Blemish Prone

If you're suffering from acne, look for serums with salicylic acid or benzoyl peroxide to help dry up blemishes and reduce inflammation on the skin that's prone to breakouts. Salicylic acid is also great for removing built-up oil in the pores, leading to unsightly blackheads or white bumps.

Anti-Redness

If your skin is easily irritated, look for calming ingredients like mint extract, aloe vera juice, and witch hazel in the ingredient list of your serum. These serums are designed not only to soothe irritation but also to minimize redness and reduce the size of any breakouts that may form under the skin.

Eye Creams

While not technically a serum, eye creams are another product designed to deliver targeted ingredients into specific areas of your face. It's best to avoid products with potentially harmful ingredients like retinol or glycolic acid around the sensitive area of your eyes.

Retinoids are one of the few exceptions because they help reduce puffiness and dark circles under the eyes while also reducing fine lines around that area. Eye creams can be used both morning and night, but be sure to avoid using them around your mouth as the product could end up in the delicate tissue of the skin and cause irritation.

How to Use a Serum in Your Skin Care Regime

Serums are the next step in your skin care routine after cleanser, toner, and moisturizer. Serums can be used on their own or with other products to target specific skin care concerns such as acne, wrinkles, dark spots, and fine lines. Some serums also help with collagen production, which helps slow down aging by keeping skin firm, smooth and healthy.

Serums are typically lightweight in consistency, making them a perfect companion to moisturizing during the skin care routine. They can be used together without feeling too heavy or greasy on your face. The exception would be serums that contain oils such as rosehip seed oil, which is very nourishing.

DIY Face Serum Recipes

Serums are concentrated products that act deep within the layers of the epidermis. They deliver nutrients and ingredients directly to different parts of your skin, making them incredibly beneficial for all types--especially dry or aging skin.

Here are some homemade face serum recipes you can make:

Face Serum for Normal Skin

The essential oils used in this recipe will help restore balance to your skin and protect it from pollutants leading to damage. Jojoba oil and Sunflower Seed Oil are very effective on normal skin types.

Ingredients:
- ¼ cup Sunflower Seed Oil (Or use Jojoba Oil)
- 15 drops Lavender Essential Oil
- 12 drops Frankincense Essential Oil
- A few drops of Vitamin E oil

Directions:
1. Combine all ingredients in a dark glass dropper bottle.
2. Shake well before each use to blend the oils together.
3. Use twice daily on clean skin using a cotton ball or facial brush for best results.

Face Serum for Oily Skin

This serum is very effective at keeping oil production under control while also soothing redness and irritation. The ingredients in this recipe give the skin a matte appearance. Use Grapeseed Oil, Tamanu Oil, or Apricot Kernel Oil as carriers.

Ingredients:
- ½ cup Grapeseed Oil or Tamanu Oil (or Apricot Kernel)
- 5 drops Lemon Essential Oil
- 3 drops of Vitamin E oil

Directions:

1. Combine all ingredients in a dark glass dropper bottle. Shake well before each use to blend the oils together.

2. Lemon essential oil is photosensitive, so avoid applying it to your skin if you intend to be out in the sun. Instead, apply it before going to bed.

3. Face Serum for Acne-Prone Skin

This face serum is designed to help soothe irritation, redness, and inflammation. It also contains ingredients that will help fight acne-causing bacteria. The tea tree oil found in this face serum is also an antiseptic. Argan Oil helps skin that is prone to breakouts.

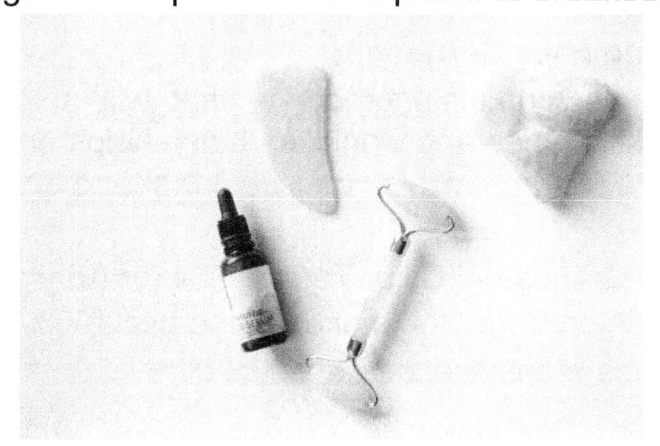

Ingredients:
- ¼ cup Aloe Vera Gel (make sure to use 100% pure aloe)
- 2 tablespoons of Argan Oil
- 5-7 drops of tea tree essential oil
- ½ Vitamin E capsule or a few drops of Vitamin E Oil

Directions:

1. Combine all ingredients in a dark glass dropper bottle, and use daily on clean skin.

Face Serum for Dry Skin

Use Rosehip Seed Oil, Sweet Almond Oil, or Avocado Oil for dry skin. This face serum will help regenerate new skin cells and keep your skin hydrated without leaving it greasy or heavy.

Ingredients:
- ½ cup Rosehip Seed Oil, Sweet Almond Oil, or Avocado Oil (or a combination)
- 15 drops of Lavender Essential oil
- A few drops of Vitamin E oil

Directions:
1. Combine all ingredients in a dark glass dropper bottle.
2. Shake well before each use to blend the oils together.
3. Use before bedtime when you want to give your skin a boost of hydration.

Anti-Aging Face Serum

This face serum contains ingredients that will help diminish the appearance of fine lines and wrinkles. It also helps protect your skin from free radical damage, which causes premature aging.

Ingredients:
- ¼ cup Grapeseed Oil or Tamanu Oil (or Apricot Kernel)
- ½ cup Aloe Vera Gel (make sure to use 100% pure aloe)
- 20 drops Frankincense Essential oil

Directions:
1. Mix well and use daily on clean skin.
2. Combine all ingredients in a dark glass dropper bottle.
3. Shake well before each use to blend the oils together.
4. Use a cotton ball or facial brush twice daily on clean skin for best results.

This face serum can be used in different combinations to address your skin care needs and concerns! Use the serum recipes mentioned above, or feel free to experiment with blends of oils that work for you.

Face Masks

Face masks are a great way to give your skin an extra boost of hydration. They also help remove dead skin cells and improve the

appearance of fine lines and wrinkles.
Masks are best used once or twice a week.

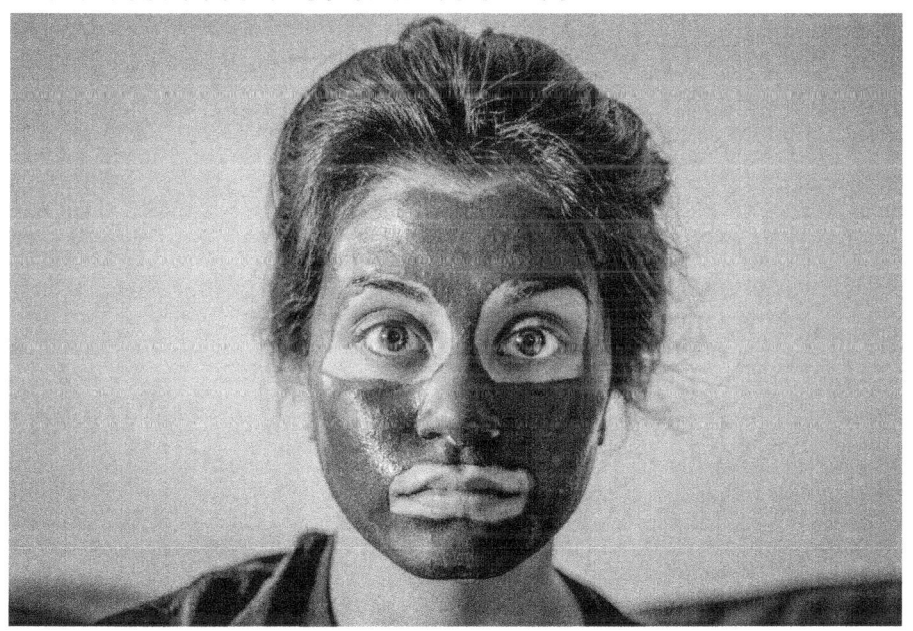

Benefits of Using a Face Mask

Here is some additional information on why you should incorporate face masks in your skin care routine:
- Removes blackheads, dirt, and oil from pores
- It helps get rid of acne
- Improves the appearance of age spots
- It helps reduce fine lines and wrinkles
- It gives skin a healthy glow by making it softer, smoother, and more radiant-looking.

How to Use a Face Mask

There are several different types of face masks that you can use. Masks should be applied to clean skin and left on for about 20 minutes before washing off with warm water.

Masks for Different Skin Ailments

Masks can address different skin concerns, including dryness and dehydration, age spots, dull skin tone, and acne-prone skin.

There are many different types of masks and recipes you can make at home.

Banana Based Face Masks

Banana is a natural source of vitamins A, B, and C. It also contains potassium which helps improve skin complexion by stimulating blood flow.

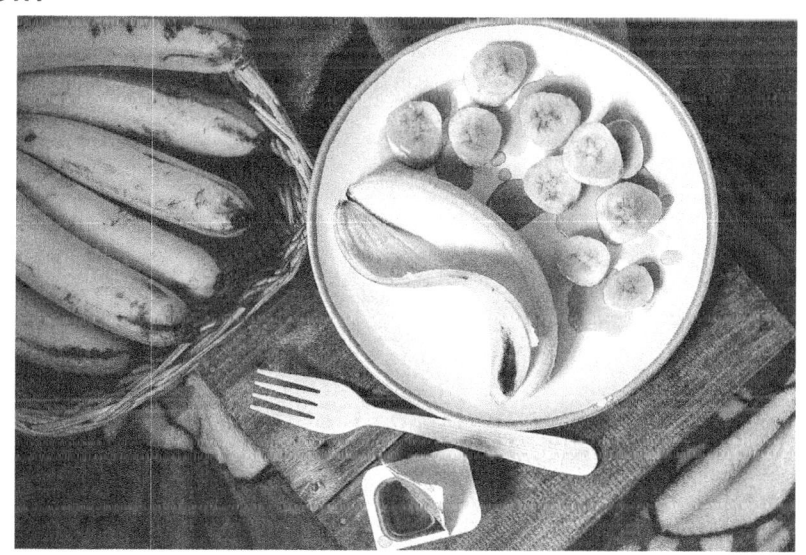

Ingredients:
- ½ Banana (mashed)

Directions:
1. Mix in a small bowl until you get a smooth paste consistency.
2. Apply to your face and neck, and leave it on for about 15 minutes before rinsing with warm water.

Apple Cider Vinegar Based Face Masks

Apple cider vinegar has been used for centuries to heal different skin ailments. It contains minerals and vitamins, which help remove dead cells from the surface of your face while stimulating blood flow into the pores.

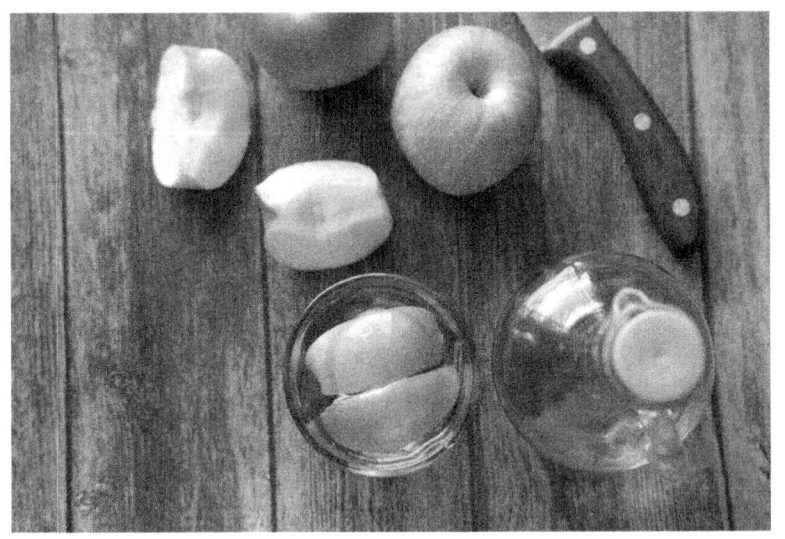

Ingredients:
- ½ cup Apple Cider Vinegar
- 1/2 cup Water

Directions:
1. Mix in a small bowl and use immediately.
2. Apply to your face with cotton balls or a facial brush for best results.
3. Let it sit for 20 minutes before rinsing off with cool water.

Milk-Based Face Masks

Milk is high in lactic acid, which helps remove dead skin cells. It also contains minerals and vitamins that help improve the appearance of your skin by making it soft, smooth, and hydrated.

Ingredients:
- ½ cup Water
- 1/2 cup Milk Powder

Directions:
1. Mix in a small bowl until you get a smooth consistency.
2. Apply to your face and leave on for about 15 minutes before rinsing with cool water.

Enhance the Benefits of Your Masks with Essential Oils

You can enhance the benefits of masks by adding essential oils. Essential oils come from plants and trees, and each one has unique benefits for your skin.

Acne-Prone Skin Masks

Add tea tree or lavender essential oils to your face mask recipes if you suffer from acne. Tea tree oil can help reduce the size of pimples and get rid of blackheads while reducing inflammation and redness in the area. Lavender essential oil is known for its antibacterial properties, reducing acne and preventing future breakouts.

Dry Skin Masks

Add rosehip seed or coconut oil to your face mask recipes if you have dry skin. Rosehip seed has antioxidants that help protect the cells of your skin while increasing collagen production. Coconut oil also helps increase collagen production and protect the cells from free radical damage. It's great for hydrating dry or ashy skin.

Age Spots Masks

Add carrot seed essential oil to your face mask recipes if you have age spots. Carrot seed has anti-inflammatory properties which help reduce redness caused by age spots. It also contains beta-carotene, which helps brighten the skin and improve elasticity, making fine lines less noticeable.

Oily Skin Masks

Add tea tree or geranium essential oils to your face mask recipes if you have oily skin. Tea tree oil can help balance out excess sebum production, which can help reduce oiliness. Geranium essential oil is known for its astringent properties, which help tighten up the skin and shrink pores to prevent breakouts from happening in the future.

Dull Skin Masks

Add lemon or grapefruit seed extract to your face mask recipes if you have dull or lackluster skin. Lemon has astringent properties, which help tighten the skin and remove dead cells from its surface. The grapefruit seed extract is known for its anti-inflammatory effects and its ability to increase collagen production in your skin, which can improve the elasticity of your facial muscles.

Itchy Skin Masks

If you have sensitive or itchy skin, it's a good idea to add lavender or chamomile essential oils to your face mask recipes. Lavender is known for its anti-inflammatory properties, which can reduce itching and irritation in the area. Chamomile has been used as a natural calmative for hundreds of years. It is great in reducing redness, itchiness, and inflammation associated with skin conditions such as eczema or psoriasis.

Some Common Ingredients Used for Masks

Clay Mask

This mask contains bentonite clay, kaolin powder, or French green clay, which helps absorb oil without drying out the skin too much. Clay also helps pull impurities from pores when it dries onto your skin. Mix two equal parts of apple cider vinegar (or coconut milk) with Bentonite clay until it forms a paste. Then add in enough filtered water to make the mixture spreadable but not runny. Add essential oils if desired, as this will give an added boost of benefits! Apply the mask evenly over your face, avoiding the eye area, and let it dry for about 20 minutes before removing it with warm water.

Sugar Mask

This mask contains ingredients like brown sugar or coconut oil which help exfoliate dead skin cells and cleanse pores by drawing out impurities when mixed together. Combine equal parts of Brown Sugar and or Coconut Oil, then add filtered water until you get a spreadable paste. Add essential oils if desired, as this will give it an added boost! Apply the mask evenly over your face, avoiding the eye areas. Let it dry for about 20 minutes, then wash off gently in the shower or sink. Pat dry with a soft towel before applying moisturizer afterward.

Clay and Egg White Masks

For this mask, combine an egg white with Bentonite clay to make a paste. Egg whites contain proteins that help tighten pores and reduce oiliness. Mix everything in a bowl and spread over your entire facial area (avoiding eye areas). Leave on for about 20 minutes, then remove by washing with warm water thoroughly.

Citrus Masks

This mask contains ingredients like lemon juice, orange peels, or grapefruit that act as natural astringents to cleanse pores and leave skin looking fresh and radiant when applied topically. Mix equal parts of raw organic honey with filtered water until the consistency is spreadable. Add essential oils if desired, as they will give added benefits! Apply the mask evenly over your face (avoiding eye areas). Then wash it off thoroughly with warm water.

Oatmeal Mask

This mask contains ingredients like ground oatmeal, green tea, or honey, which help soothe the skin when applied topically and provide anti-inflammatory benefits to reduce redness from acne breakouts. Combine equal parts of organic raw honey with filtered water until you get a spreadable paste. Add essential oils if desired; they will give added benefits! Mix in ground oatmeal, then apply the mixture onto clean skin, avoid the eye area, and let it dry for about 20 minutes. Rinse well and pat dry before applying moisturizer afterward.

Important Considerations While Using Serums and Face Masks

Serums are generally more effective than face masks. They penetrate the skin deeper and seep into its pores, allowing for better absorption of ingredients to nourish your skin cells.

Serums also tend to contain higher concentrations of active ingredients like vitamins which can help combat signs of aging or other external factors that may cause problems with your complexion. Some serums need specific types of creams to work properly. These products should be used together at night before you head off to bed, so they have time to get absorbed by the body's natural processes while it rests.

If you're looking for a good serum-cream combination, try using one containing Vitamin C along with an anti-aging cream made from Retinol or Retinoids. Retinol is a form of Vitamin A that has been shown to improve skin texture and appearance over time. Retinoids are more powerful and can help reduce signs of aging like fine lines and wrinkles by stimulating collagen production in your cells.

Some face masks also contain serums as an important ingredient. However, people looking for anti-aging properties should look for a product containing AHAs or Alpha Hydroxy Acids, which help remove dead layers from the epidermis (the outermost layer), where most dryness occurs due to exposure to sunlight.

This process helps reveal smoother and younger-looking skin underneath; however, make sure not to rub it too hard to avoid irritating your skin.

Masks containing AHAs can also help remove signs of hyperpigmentation (brown spots and patches that appear on the face due to sun exposure or hormonal changes) which is a common problem among women over 30, especially if they have darker complexions.

Shelf Life of DIY Skin Care Products

If you are using natural or organic products, always use your best judgment for how long it will last before the product degrades in quality and effectiveness. Many factors affect this, including changing seasons, heat exposure, storage location, etc.

Here are a few general rules:

- Oils have an indefinite shelf life if stored properly, and it's even possible to cook with old oils. You can test them by smelling them first, and as long as they smell fine, they should be okay.
- H20-Based Toners and Mists must be kept refrigerated at all times to prevent bacterial growth.
- Milk and Cleansers must be kept refrigerated at all times.
- Balms, Butters and Balm-Like DIYs will stay for up to two years if stored in a cool dark place away from sunlight. Suppose your balm comes with oil like argan or almond. In that case, it'll last even longer because the oil has natural antimicrobial properties that act as preservatives.
- Solid butter can also sometimes melt during hot weather, so it should be kept out of direct heat too. Just pop them back into the fridge until firm again if you want them solidified.

Serums and masks are a great way to give your skin that extra boost of moisture, which will help it feel suppler. They also have the added benefit of helping with wrinkles!

And that's it! We hope this has helped you understand how to use serums and masks properly in your skin care routine. Serums are great for brightening the skin, while masks help with firming or moisturizing. You can even mix them and make a super-moisturizing mask serum.

Chapter 6: Yummy Body Butters

In this chapter, we will explore the idea of adding body butter to your skin care routine. We will discuss what they are, how they differ from lotions and other moisturizers, and why it is important to include them in your routine. We will also provide a few recipes for making yummy body butter at home!

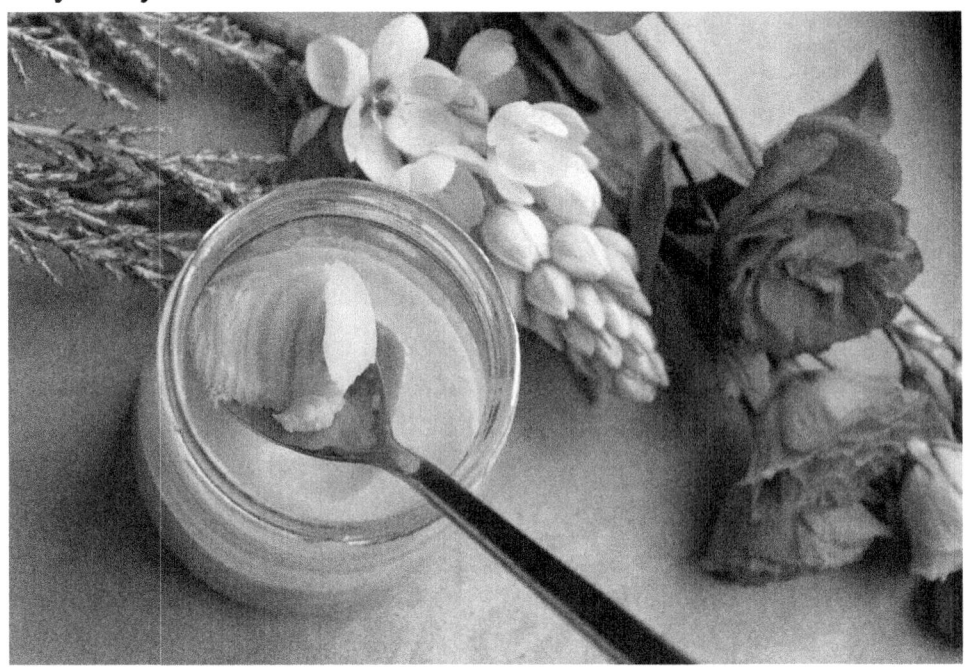

What Is Body Butter?

Body butter is super-rich and thick moisturizers designed to be used on the body. They contain a higher percentage of water than lotions and several oils such as cocoa butter or shea butter that provide emollient properties for softening skin. Body butter may also include other ingredients like glycerin, aloe vera, vitamin E, and more!

How Do Body Butters Differ from Lotions?

While lotions are generally lighter in texture than butter, they often contain fewer oils. This is why some people feel that body butter can be better for skin health because it may provide a deeper level of moisture. However, it's essential to keep in mind that lotions are more convenient to apply after a shower because they get absorbed quickly. At the same time, body butter may leave your skin feeling oily if you don't pat it dry.

When Should You Use Body Butters?

Body butter can be used year-round. However, there is a bit of extra hydration benefit during winters. You can use them after a shower, but they are also great to layer under a thicker moisturizer if the temperatures drop and skin starts feeling dry!

Recipes for Body Butters

Here are some of our favorite recipes that you can easily make at home with lovely scents or ingredients that can be found around the house:

Cinnamon Vanilla Body Butter

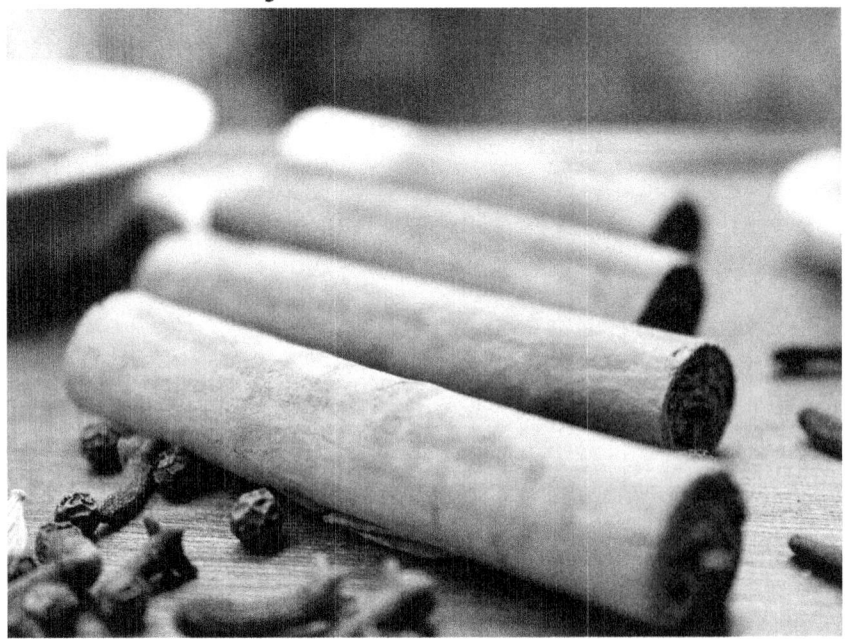

Ingredients:
- 15g Cocoa Butter (0.5 oz) (can also use shea)
- 20 drops of Vanilla Essential Oil or preferred scent (try our organic lavender!)
- 40ml oils (1.3 oz), can be Olive/Almond/Jojoba, etc. We prefer a mix of a few different oils.
- **Optional**: 20 drops Cinnamon Essential Oil

Directions:

1. Put the cocoa butter/ shea butter in a microwave-safe bowl. Melt for 30 seconds at a time until completely melted. We recommend using a double boiler to melt the

butter. However, if you are in a hurry or don't have access to it, you can go ahead and microwave.

2. Once melted, turn off the stove. Combine oils (this is best done by pouring them slowly into another bowl while whisking) and add essential oil(s). At this point, you can also add cinnamon oil if you would like a wonderful autumn scent!

3. Mix everything and pour into a jar or container. This recipe yields approximately 100ml of body butter, enough for around two months, depending on how often it is used. We recommend storing the butter in a cool place, like your fridge or a cool, dark cupboard.

4. You can also make larger quantities of this recipe and pour it into an empty lotion container, making them perfect gifts.

Tropical Body Butter

This body butter smells like a tropical vacation!

Ingredients:

- 100ml Olive Oil (3 oz) (or any other carrier oils you like to use)
- 15g Cocoa Butter (0.5 oz)(can also use shea)
- 20 drops of Coconut Essential Oil *optional*

Directions:

1. Follow the same steps as above.

2. Coconut oil has a rich, nutty scent that will turn this body butter into something tropical and extraordinary! Suppose you don't have essential coconut oil. In that case, you can either replace it with vanilla or another scented oil of your choice.

Honey Vanilla Body Butter

Honey and Vanilla are a classic combination, and this body butter is sure to make your skin feel extra yummy. Honey is also a humectant, so it is great for locking in moisture.

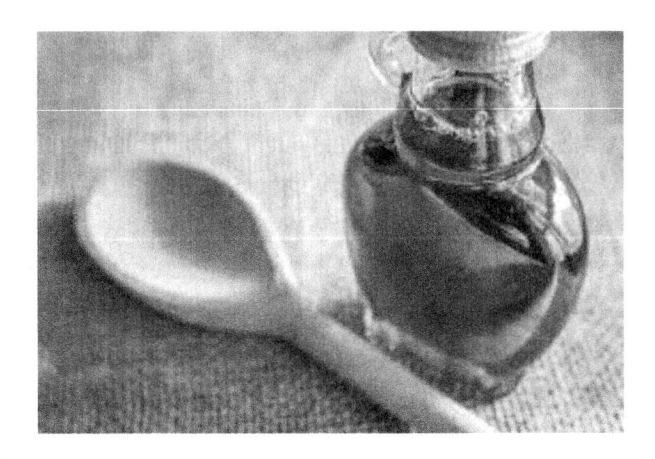

Ingredients:

- 40g Shea or Cocoa Butter (around one ounce), You can also use a mix of the butter if you like!
- 15g Coconut Oil
- 20 drops of Vanilla Essential Oil
- 15g Honey (0.45 oz) or a couple of teaspoons if you have a drippy consistency in mind!
- **Optional**: Add some beeswax for extra hold and texture; around 0.75oz will be enough for this recipe. If using beeswax, make sure to heat it first and then add to the oils.
- **Optional:** A few drops of your favorite colorant (we like using beetroot powder or spinach for natural coloring)

Directions:

1. Melt shea/cocoa butter and coconut oil together in a double boiler on low heat until melted.
2. Remove from the stovetop, mix in desired essential oil(s) and colorant.
3. Add the honey at the end and blend it in.

Vanilla Bean Body Butter

This body butter is great to use when you need something a little thicker and creamier. Using 100% shea butter in this recipe would make for an incredibly rich moisturizer that might be too thick for some people, but feel free to experiment with different ratios, depending on your skin type.

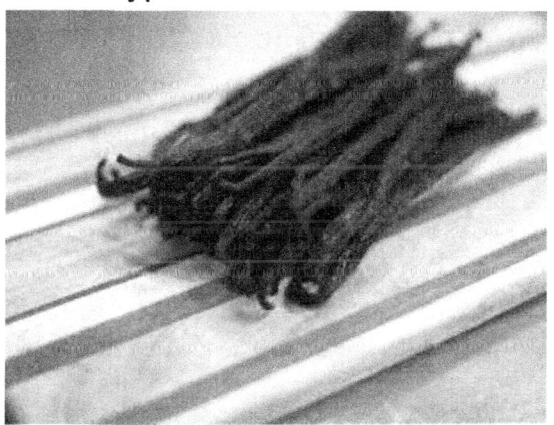

Ingredients:
- 1 cup raw Cocoa Butter
- 1/2 cup Sweet Almond Oil
- 1/2 cup Coconut Oil
- 1 Vanilla Bean

Directions:
1. Heat the cocoa butter and coconut oil in a double boiler until melted. Remove from heat, add in the ground vanilla bean, cover for about 15 minutes to let the flavors infuse, and mix in the almond oil.

2. Keep it in the freezer until the oils solidify, and then whip the body butter with a hand mixer until light, fluffy and smooth. Store in an airtight container or jar.

3. You can also add different essential oils based on your preference; lavender is great if you have trouble sleeping! Rosemary has mood-boosting properties that may help improve your mood when you're feeling low.

Whipped Coconut Oil Body Butter
This body butter is a great alternative if you are looking for something that feels lighter and absorbs more quickly into the skin.

Ingredients:
- 1 cup Coconut Oil
- 1 teaspoon Vitamin E Oil (optional)
- Your Favorite Essential Oil- A few drops of your chosen essential oil per tablespoon of coconut oil is a good rule of thumb.

Directions:

1. In a bowl, whip the coconut oil until light and fluffy.
2. Mix in the desired amount of essential oils and vitamin E, then transfer into jars or containers for storage.

Whipped Peppermint Body Butter

This whipped moisturizer has a cooling, refreshing effect that is both energizing and relaxing at the same time! The peppermint essential oil also makes it great to use in the morning when you need an extra boost of energy.

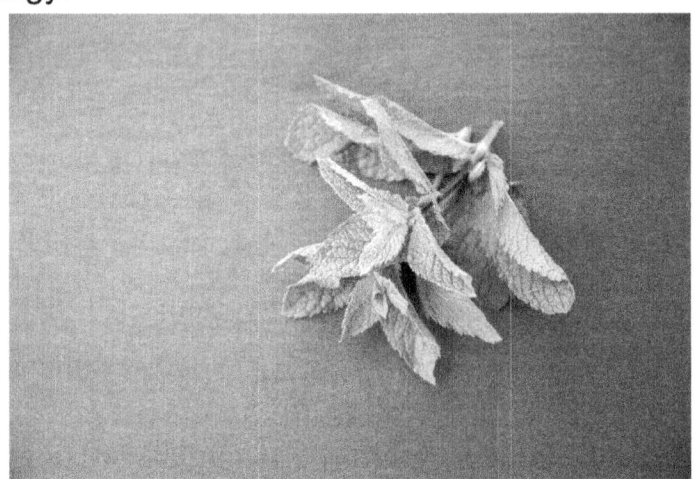

Ingredients:
- 1 cup Shea Butter or Cocoa Butter
- 25 drops of Peppermint Essential Oil
- ***Optional:*** Add some beeswax for extra hold and texture; around 0.75oz will be enough for this recipe. If using beeswax, make sure you heat it first and then add it to the oils.

Directions:
1. Melt the shea/cocoa butter in a double boiler until melted.
2. Remove from heat, add the desired amount of essential peppermint oil and transfer to jars or containers for storage.

Honey Almond Body Butter

This body butter is great for when you need something light and nourishing. It gets absorbed quickly into the skin without leaving an oily residue behind! The honey will also help to keep your skin soft, smooth, and hydrated.

Ingredients:
- 1 cup almond oil
- 1/3rd cup coconut oil
- 1/5 cup raw honey (around a couple of teaspoons if you have a drippy consistency in mind!
- A few drops of your favorite essential oil; we recommend lavender or lemon for a relaxing effect in the evening and peppermint if you want something more refreshing in the morning.

Directions:
1. Melt coconut oil and almond oil in a double boiler on low heat until melted. Remove from heat and transfer to another bowl. Let the oil mixture cool until it starts to solidify, usually for about an hour at normal room temperature.
2. Once cooled, whip with a hand mixer or by hand until light and fluffy (about 15 minutes). Add in the desired amount of essential oils and honey and whisk/mix together well! Transfer to jars or containers for storage.
3. This body butter is great to use after the shower, especially if you want something that will lock in the moisture and leave your skin feeling silky smooth throughout the day! It can be a bit hard to spread on dry areas of your skin, so we recommend

applying it while you're still damp after stepping out of the shower.

Making your own body butter and other moisturizing products is a wonderful way to experiment with new scents. Get creative and try something you've always wanted to make! It's also fairly easy once you know what you are doing. We recommend starting small by making one recipe at a time until it becomes second nature.

Body Butters with Specific Properties
Chapped Skin/Eczema

If you have problematic skin that is dry and/or gets chapped quickly, body butter with cocoa butter is a great solution. Cocoa butter has properties that allow it to penetrate deeper into the outer layer of the skin while locking in moisture simultaneously. This makes them ideal for people who suffer from eczema or any other conditions that cause the skin to be dry and itchy.

Acne-Prone Skin

If you have skin prone to breakouts, body butters with shea butter and/or coconut oil can be a great addition to your morning or night-time regimens. Shea butter has anti-inflammatory properties that help reduce redness and swelling while also penetrating deep into the upper layers of the epidermis!

Coconut oil is also great for reducing inflammation and redness and nourishing the skin to keep it hydrated.

Stretch Marks

For recent stretch marks or the ones still in the early stages, body butter with cocoa butter can be an incredible addition! Cocoa butter has properties that allow it to penetrate deep into the upper layer of the epidermis, which can help reduce the appearance of stretch marks over time.

Suppose you are looking to prevent stretch marks during pregnancy or existing stretch marks that are still fresh. In that case, body butter with shea butter and/or cocoa butter are a great option! Shea butter has anti-inflammatory properties that can help reduce redness and swelling while also allowing it to penetrate deep into the upper layers of the epidermis.

Stretch marks that are already a little deeper can also benefit from shea butter. Cocoa butter is great at reducing the appearance of stretch marks over time.

Cellulite/Sagging Skin

If you have skin that has lost its elasticity and firmness due to age or weight loss, body butter made with shea butter is a great choice. Shea butter has anti-inflammatory properties that can help ease the pain of sore, stiff, or tired muscles while also nourishing your skin to keep it hydrated and looking healthy.

Shea Butter is one of the most emollient plant butters known to man. It is great for dry, cracked skin and works well with other ingredients due to its thick consistency.

Best Essential Oil Combinations for Body Butter

Peppermint and lavender are probably the most common essential oil combinations for body butter.

Not only does it smell incredible, but peppermint has a cooling effect that makes it great to use in the morning while lavender is calming and relaxing at night time.

If you want something with an earthy scent, try pairing patchouli and sandalwood, as both have a more woodsy aroma.

If you prefer something fruity, lemon and orange essential oil will do the trick.

Add cinnamon, clove, or nutmeg if you want to add a little extra kick! Frankincense and myrrh are also excellent essential oils to use in combination with other ingredients.

Gingerbread Spice Combination

This is a great combination to make your body butter smell like gingerbread cookies. Add in some nutmeg, clove, lemon, and orange essential oil for the ultimate winter scent!

Lavender-Gingerbread Spice Combination

If lavender isn't your favorite, then try out this combination instead. Add in some gingerbread essential oil, lemon, and orange for the perfect holiday blend.

Coconut-Lavender Combination

This is a great combination if you like the scent of lavender and want to add in some extra moisturizing properties with coconut oil. The smell isn't too overpowering, so it will work well for those who prefer something subtle. Add in your favorite essential oils for an even stronger scent.

Coconut-Peppermint Combination

This is the perfect combination if you want a cooling effect, ideal to use in the morning time! Add peppermint essential oil into your mixture before microwaving it, along with coconut oil and shea butter. This will give you that refreshing smell and is also great for the skin.

Coconut-Gingerbread Spice Combination

This combination has a strong scent that is perfect to use during the winter. Try adding some gingerbread essential oil and nutmeg, clove, or cinnamon into your mixture after microwaving it with coconut oil and shea butter. Now you have a body butter that smells just like gingerbread!

Coconut-Frankincense and Myrrh Combination

This is another great combination if you want something that has an earthy, woodsy scent.

Unscented Combination

If you are sensitive to strong smells or prefer something with no scent at all, then try out this simple but effective combination. Combine shea butter, coconut oil, and cocoa butter into one bowl before microwaving (in 20-second increments) and stirring until it is completely melted. This mixture has a very mild organic smell and will not trigger any allergies or sensitivities.

Try pairing your body butter with some bath salts for a luxurious gift. Add lavender and/or peppermint essential oils to the mix before transferring them into jars for gifting. See how easy it can be?

Shelf Life for Homemade Body Butters

If stored in a dry, cool place, body butter should last up to three months.

If stored in a somewhat warm place, body butters can melt because of their oils.

If this happens, place the container in the refrigerator to harden it up. Make sure that it is properly sealed so that no water gets into the mixture. If you have kids at home, it is best to keep the body butter in a safe place out of their reach.

Lotions are different from body butter because they contain water-based ingredients instead of oils. This makes lotions lighter and less moisturizing than body butter, which is why it's important to have both in your skin care routine!

How to Use a Body Butter in Your Skin Care Routine

Body butter can be used in place of lotion or as a moisturizer after you cleanse and tone your skin. Take some body butter onto your hands and rub them together before applying it to the desired area of your face, neck, and even décolleté.

You should always apply any skincare product to damp skin because that is when the product will be most effective.

Pour some body butter into your hands and then use them to massage it onto your neck gently, face (avoiding contact with eyes), and décolleté in circular motions for about one minute. This process allows the butters time to penetrate deep within your pores so that you get maximum moisturizing benefits.

If your skin feels tight or dry after cleansing, use body butter to give yourself an extra boost of moisture.

Should You Use a Lotion, Moisturizer, or Body Butter?

That all depends on your preference.

Lotions are light and not greasy at all, moisturizers can be a bit too heavy for some people, but they get absorbed quickly into the skin. Body butter is known to have a thicker consistency that stays longer compared to lotions or moisturizers. It also has heavier ingredients which provide maximum moisturizing benefits.

Different Types of Body Butters to Try Out

Try experimenting with different ingredients to find your favorite combination perfect for your skin type and needs.

Coconut Oil-Shea Butter Combination

This is a great body butter if you have dry, flaky, or itchy skin. The coconut oil and shea butter moisturize the skin very well while protecting it from environmental damage that leads to premature aging or irritation.

Shea Butter-Cocoa Butter Combination

This is a very thick mixture, but if you have really sensitive, dry skin, then this will become your best friend! Shea butter contains lauric acid, which can help clear away acne, and cocoa butter is an excellent moisturizer that also contains antioxidants.

Coconut Oil-Jojoba Oil Combination

This body butter has a lot of slip to it, making it perfect for giving your skin some extra moisture but without feeling too greasy or heavy. Jojoba is a great oil that closely resembles the natural oils of our skin!

Vitamin E-Coconut Oil Combination

This is one of my favorites, especially in the summer when it's hot out. Vitamin E is an antioxidant that can help protect your skin from sun damage, and coconut oil has many benefits and keeps your skin looking youthful and glowing.

Considerations before Using a Body Butter

It is important to check ingredients and make sure that you are not allergic to any.

Do a patch test to determine if you have any sensitivities or allergies. Apply a small amount of body butter to your forearm and wait for 24 hours before using it on the rest of your body.

If, after waiting for a total of 24 hours, there are no signs of redness, irritation, or itching, then congratulations! You can use that combination without worrying about an allergic reaction.

If you do have an allergic reaction, stop using the body butter immediately!

If your skin becomes irritated after using body butter, try mixing it with some coconut oil before applying it next time, or stop usage altogether if irritation persists. You can always get in touch with an esthetician for more help and guidance with creating your body butter.

We hope you found this guide on how to make DIY body butters interesting and informative. We know that there is a lot of confusion surrounding the terms "body butter," "lotion," and "cream," so we wanted to clarify what they are and why it matters when choosing skincare products for your routine. Creating these recipes at home involves only two-three ingredients (and sometimes fewer), which can be bought in bulk or purchased from natural food stores as per your requirements. If you want some more ideas on organic alternatives for harsh chemicals used in cosmetics, read on…

Chapter 7: Organic Lotions and Balms

It is a known fact that the skin is our largest organ. It was not until recently that we have been able to fully appreciate all of its functions, one being to produce needed oil for itself. This oil moisturizes the skin and keeps it from drying out. In this chapter, you will learn how organic lotions can help your skin stay hydrated while using natural ingredients instead of resorting to using harmful chemicals. You will also find information on how to make balm at home with recipes provided in this book!

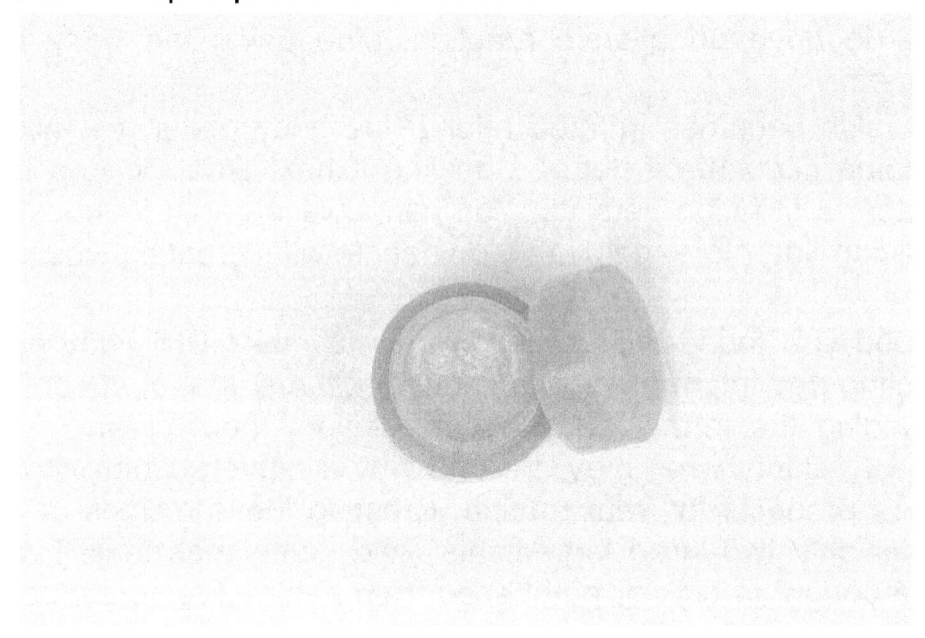

Difference between Lotions and Other Creams and Moisturizers

Lotions are lighter than most moisturizers, with creams being the thickest. Lotions penetrate the skin more quickly and get absorbed faster without leaving a greasy residue behind. They also tend to have lighter ingredients, so they may not give you as much of an overall moisturizing effect but can still help maintain hydration. On the other hand, creams are thicker and have more oil, so they tend to last longer than lotions with a similar amount of product used.

Lotions work best for people who have sensitive or acne-prone skin because they typically contain lighter ingredients that won't clog pores as easily as other moisturizers might.

Another difference between creams and lotions is that the latter are mostly water-based, while creams or balms are oil-based. You can think of this as being similar to how olive oil is thicker than water, so it doesn't mix very well. However, new technologies have been able to combine these two ingredients into one product, with positive results.

What Is a Balm, and How Is It Different from Creams and Lotions?

If you use a moisturizer to help your skin look fresh and healthy, then you're most likely aware of these three types: creams, lotions, and balms. But how do they differ from each other? Which type is best for your face or body? We have broken down the differences between these popular skincare products so you can choose the moisturizer best suited for your skin type.

Creams are ideal for dry, sensitive skin because they have a thicker consistency and often contain more natural ingredients than lotions or balms.

Lotions are more suitable for oily and combination skins because they have a lighter consistency and can be absorbed into the skin quickly.

Solidified oils that melt when they get in touch with your skin's heat are called skin balms. Balms do not contain water and provide a more robust shield for your skin to protect it from external elements such as dry, cold air. Balms are usually the final step in a skin care routine.

Lotions

Lotions should be applied after a shower when the skin is damp, as it allows better absorption.

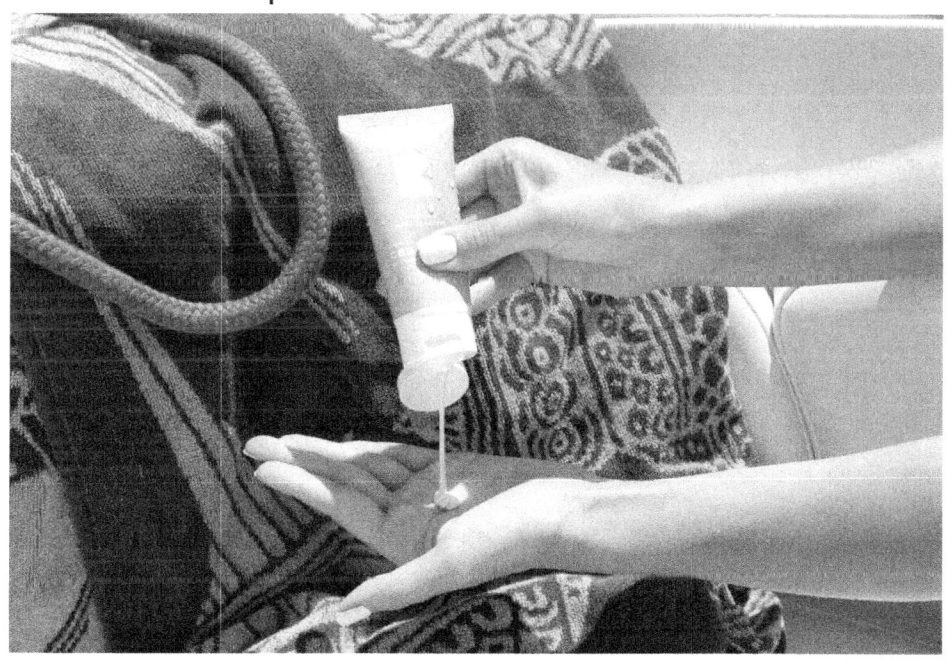

Lotions should be applied all over the body - including areas that rub together, such as inner thighs and underarms. This prevents rashes from developing in these delicate places where creams may not absorb well enough to provide relief.

Many people have combination skin, which means their face is dry while other parts of the body are oily. If you have this type of skin, it's best to use a cream on your whole body, with the exception of your face.

If you get lotion in any cuts or scrapes that may develop from shaving, apply antibiotic ointment over the area.

Lotions that contain SPF (sun protection factor) are best for people who like to spend their time in the sun, as they will protect your skin from harmful UV rays. If you're not a big fan of outdoor activities and rarely find yourself under direct sunlight, it's okay to use a lotion without an SPF on most parts of the body.

DIY Organic Lotion Recipes

We've got you covered with some easy-to-make organic lotion recipes.

Almond Rose Night Lotion

Almond is one of the most nourishing oils, and rose water is great for dry skin.

Ingredients:
- 1/4 cup Almond Oil
- ½ Teaspoon Vitamin E oil or Vitamin E powder
- ½ cup Rose Water
- 1 Tablespoon Beeswax
- ¼ cup Coconut Oil

Expert Tip*: Add honey to the mixture for a nice smell and a binding effect*

Directions:

1. Mix almond oil and vitamin E in a mixing bowl until well combined.

2. Put rose water, beeswax, and coconut oil into a saucepan or a double boiler over low heat just until the wax is melted. Remove from the heat immediately to avoid burning it. Let it cool for about 30 seconds before adding to the oil mixture, then stir quickly so as not to cool too much.

3. Warm the rose water a little before pouring it into the mixture to blend well.

4. Store in a clean, airtight jar.

Shea Butter and Honey Lotion

Shea butter is widely used to treat skin conditions such as dermatitis, eczema, scars, and stretch marks. It absorbs well into the skin without leaving a greasy feeling behind. Plus, it has anti-inflammatory properties too!

Ingredients:

- ¼th cup Shea Butter (melted)
- ¼th cup Cocoa Butter (melted)
- ½ teaspoon of Vitamin E Oil or Vitamin E powder
- ½ - ¾th cup Almond Oil (Use more for dry skin, less for normal/oily skin types)

Directions:

1. Melt Shea and cocoa butter in a double boiler.

2. Remove from heat and add Vitamin E oil or powder, almond oil, and honey to the mixture while it's still warm. Stir well until ingredients are well blended. Pour into a jar or container with an airtight lid for storage.

Shea Butter and Olive Oil Lotion

Olive oil is rich in antioxidants that help fight off free radicals that can lead to skin damage. It's also great for preventing dryness of the skin.

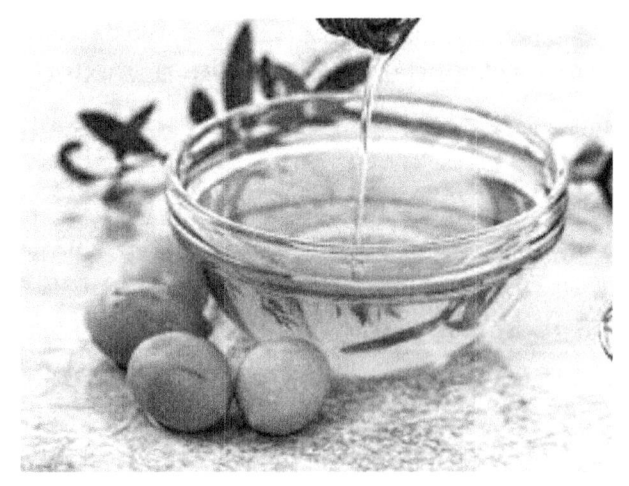

Ingredients:

- ½ cup Shea Butter (melted)
- ¼ cup Olive Oil

Directions:

1. Melt Shea Butter in a double boiler.

2. Remove from heat and add Olive oil to the mixture while it's still warm; stir well until ingredients are blended thoroughly.

3. Pour into an airtight container for storage.

Lotion for Oily Skin

Oily skin types can go for a lighter lotion such as the ones above. It'll help to absorb oil and leave your skin feeling fresh all day long!

Ingredients:
- 1 cup Rose Water/distilled water/aloe vera juice
- ¼th cup Jojoba Oil or Almond Oil
- ½ cup Beeswax
- Few drops of Vitamin E

Directions:

1. Mix water, oil, and beeswax in a double boiler or glass bowl placed over simmering water.

2. Remove from heat when the wax is melted.

3. Add Vitamin E, essential oils of your choice (optional), and stir well until all ingredients are blended thoroughly.

4. Pour into an airtight jar for storage with a lid to prevent evaporation.

Shelf Life of Homemade Lotions

Since these are natural, chemical-free lotions with no added preservatives to extend shelf life, you may find that the mixture starts smelling rancid after a certain period of time.

Every homemade lotion will have its own specific shelf life depending on how quickly it absorbs into your skin and what ingredients were used to make it.

Water-based lotions will generally expire faster than oil-based ones. Storage of lotion in a dark, cool place such as your bathroom cabinet or dresser drawer may help to extend the shelf life, but do not store them under direct sunlight and never refrigerate them!

If you refrigerate a lotion, it will last longer and stay fresh.

Skin Balms

Skin balms are very popular for a reason. They are an easy, convenient way to moisturize the skin. The consistency of these balms is thicker than traditional lotions and oils, which makes them great for dry patches on elbows, knees, feet, etc.

What Is a Skin Balm?

A skin balm is a thick moisturizer with solid consistency that melts into the skin when applied.

Why Use a Skin Balm?

There are many benefits to using these balms in place of traditional lotions and oils because they offer higher concentrations of natural ingredients for maximum results. These products do not contain water which means you will get more products with a higher concentration of ingredients for a lower price.

Benefits of Using a Face Balm

Overnight Skin Repair

Skin balms and face oils work best when used overnight to repair damaged skin. Because they have a thick, heavy consistency, they can be applied before bed without worrying about excess transfer on your pillowcases.

Skin Redness

Face balms are perfect if you suffer from redness around the cheeks or nose area. Many skin balms contain ingredients like coconut oil, aloe vera, and shea butter, all-natural anti-inflammatory agents that help reduce skin redness overnight to minimize issues like rosacea or acne-related breakouts.

Sensitive Skin Care

If you have sensitive skin, these products may be a great option for you. Many of the ingredients in these balms are natural and hypoallergenic, which means they won't irritate or inflame your skin like chemical-filled products.

Skin Repair with Vitamin E

One essential vitamin that is commonly included in face balm formulations is Vitamin E. It helps to reduce redness and repair the skin after exposure to harsh conditions.

Skin Repair with Argan Oil

Argan oil is a really popular ingredient in skin balm formulations because it contains Vitamin E and fatty acids, which work to repair the skin, reduce redness, and bring balance back to your face. This makes these products perfect for reducing wrinkles around the eyes or mouth.

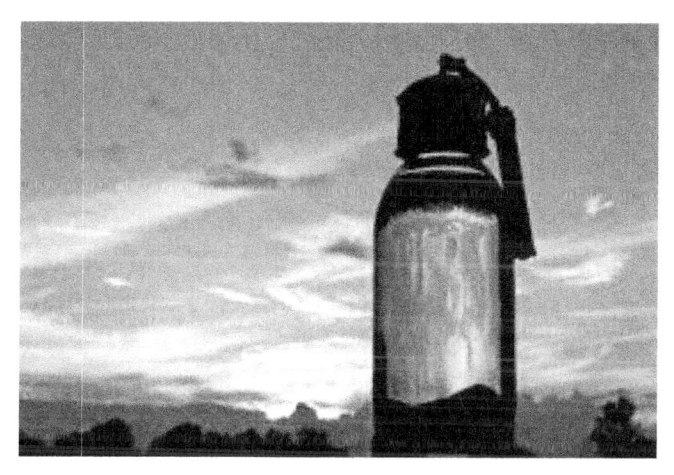

Skin Repair with Macadamia Oil

Macadamia oil is another ingredient that offers many benefits for your skin. It contains essential fatty acids which reduce inflammation and repair the skin while also containing Vitamin E, which fights off free radicals in the body! This makes it perfect for helping with signs of aging because it can slow down the damage caused by exposure to the sun and your phone's harmful rays.

How to Incorporate a Face Balm in Your Skin Care Routine

There are many ways to incorporate a face balm into your skin care routine. One of the best ways is to use it as an alternative for primer before applying foundation or concealer. These ingredients work well with makeup products and won't make them slide off throughout the day. You can also use this product after cleansing or toning while your skin is still damp to help seal in moisture and make your makeup last longer. For those with sensitive skin, you can use this product as a moisturizer at night before bed or even during the day, if needed, because these formulas tend to be thicker than traditional lotions and oils.

What Ingredients Should I Look for in a Face Balm?

There are some ingredients you should definitely look out for, like pumpkin seed oil, aloe vera, and coconut oil because they contain properties that work naturally to reduce the redness in the skin.

Other great ingredients include green tea extract, known as one of the most powerful antioxidants on earth, along with argan oil, vitamin E, and shea butter.

Oatmeal, Shea Butter, Vitamin E

The best face balms contain ingredients like oatmeal which help soothe the skin while also adding a light exfoliation for an all-around complexion boost. This ingredient is really popular in formulations because of its ability to reduce redness too! There are also other ingredients like shea butter, which help repair the skin, reduce wrinkles, and soothe irritation.

Calendula Oil

One of the best types of oil you can find in face balms is calendula oil. It contains many antioxidants that work together with Vitamin E to protect your skin against free radicals while also helping to eliminate redness and reduce inflammation.

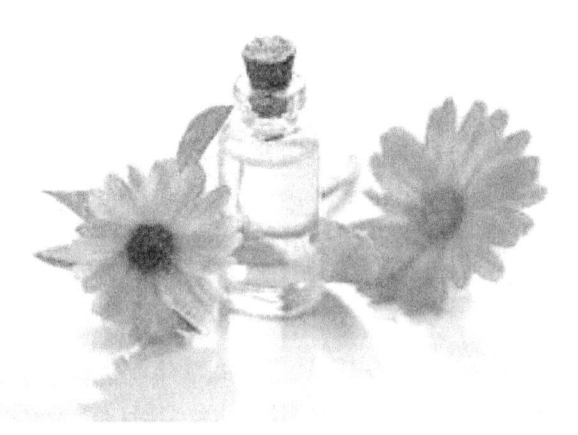

Healing and Glow Enhancing Face Balm

This is a great face balm for all skin types because it includes ingredients like hemp seed oil, rosehip seeds oil, and shea butter which help to retain moisture in the skin while also nourishing dry patches. If you have acne-prone or oily skin, this is an excellent choice because its light texture will not clog pores or leave your skin feeling greasy.

Ingredients:
- 1 tbsp Hemp Oil
- 1 tbsp Rosehip Seed Oil
- 1 tbsp Shea Butter
- 1/2 tbsp Beeswax
- 3 drops of Cypress Essential Oil
- 3 drops of Frankincense Essential Oil
- 3 drops of Bergamot Essential Oil

Directions:

1. Mix all ingredients in a glass bowl and stir until completely combined. Store the mixture in an airtight container, preferably made of glass. Apply this product after cleansing or toning your face to lock moisture into your skin.

2. Apply face balm by massaging it into your entire face, avoiding the eye area. You can use circular motions or patting motions, whatever feels most comfortable for you.

3. Wash off with water and pat dry. Exfoliate with a soft washcloth to remove dead skin cells and oil buildup.

4. You can also apply this product before applying makeup to your face as a primer, but be sure to let it fully absorb into the skin first.

Hydrating Overnight Face Balm

This face balm is great to prevent acne and repair any damage to the skin while also hydrating it with long-lasting moisture. If you struggle with redness on your face, this product could be perfect for you because its antioxidants work together to eliminate dead cells, reduce irritation, and promote new cell growth.

Rosehip oil helps repair skin damage while also reducing redness.

Lavender oil is a powerful antiseptic that works to repair skin tissue and ease inflammation, making it perfect for treating acne-prone skin without causing irritation.

Frankincense essential oil contains antioxidants that protect the skin from free radicals and reduce any signs of aging, so your face stays looking young and healthy.

Cocoa butter, Shea Butter, and Beeswax

This product is perfect for all skin types because it's lightweight but also very moisturizing due to the addition of cocoa butter, shea butter, and beeswax. It works perfectly as an overnight treatment or a mid-day face pick-me-up because its light texture won't clog your pores or leave your skin feeling greasy.

Ingredients:

- 1/4 cup Shea Butter
- 1 tbsp Cocoa Butter
- 1 1/2 tbsp Candelilla Wax
- 1/4 cup Hemp Seed Oil
- 1 tbsp Castor Oil
- 1 tbsp Rosehip Oil
- 1/2 tsp Pink Clay
- 8 drops of Geranium Essential Oil
- 8 drops of Lavender Essential Oil
- 8 drops of Frankincense Essential Oil

Directions:

1. Place all ingredients in a double boiler and stir until completely melted. Remove from heat when the mixture is fully combined with no lumps; usually, about 30 minutes of stirring on low heat will do the trick! Pour into an airtight container like glass to keep it from going rancid. Store in a dark, cool place to make the product last longer.

2. Apply this face balm by massaging it onto your entire face, avoiding the eye area, and gently rubbing any excess on your neck. You can use circular motions or patting motions, whatever feels most comfortable for you.

3. Wash off with water and pat dry. Exfoliate with a soft washcloth to remove dead skin cells and oil buildup.

Rose and Shea Face Balm

This is a great recipe for dry, sensitive, or acne-prone skin because it's so moisturizing! Rosehip oil is very high in antioxidants which are powerful at repairing skin damage and irritation while also reducing redness. Honey myrtle essential oil calms the skin down. It reduces any signs of inflammation or discomfort caused by breakouts, while geranium essential oil has astringent properties that tighten the skin and reduce pore size.

These rose, shea, and honey face balms are great for keeping your skin looking young because it reduces fine lines and wrinkles while also firming up loose or sagging skin. Rose essential oil contains vitamin C, which stimulates new cell growth, so you get a fresh layer of cells every time you use this product! Shea butter heals damaged tissue by providing moisture deep within the layers of your epidermis, where collagen production occurs naturally in younger people, making their outer layer more resilient against damage from UV rays, pollutants, etc.

Ingredients:
- 2 tablespoons Dried Rose Petals
- ¼ cup Olive Oil
- ¼ cup Shea Butter
- 2 tablespoons Beeswax
- 1 tablespoon Castor Oil or Rosehip Oil
- ½ teaspoon Australian Pink Clay
- 8 drops of Geranium Essential Oil
- 8 drops of Lavender Essential Oil

- 8 drops of Honey Myrtle Essential Oil

Directions:

1. Place all ingredients except essential oils in a double boiler over low heat until they are completely melted.

2. Remove from heat and add essential oils. Pour into a glass jar for storage.

3. Apply to your face using circular motions with the fingertips, avoiding the eye area, until the product has been absorbed by the skin.

4. Wash off with water, pat dry and massage your face lightly to exfoliate dead cells, making your pores appear smaller over time!

Cleansing Face Balm

This cleansing face balm is perfect for sensitive, acne-prone, and dry skin. It's a great option if you want to reduce the size of your pores because cocoa butter and shea butter shrink pore size while absorbing excess oil from the skin.

Coconut oil contains lauric acid, which helps kill off bacteria that causes breakouts without harming healthy cells as benzoyl peroxide does! Geranium essential oil calms inflamed or irritated skin down so it can heal quickly without any permanent damage being caused by overzealous cleaning with harsh chemicals.

Ingredients:

- 2 tablespoons Shea Butter
- 1 tablespoon Coconut Oil
- 4 Cocoa Butter Disks
- 1 teaspoon Calendula Oil
- 5 drops of Geranium Essential Oil
- 5 drops of Frankincense Essential Oil
- 5 drops of Bergamot Essential Oil

Directions:

1. Melt all ingredients, except essential oils, over a double-boiler or in a heatproof glass bowl placed inside a pot of boiling water.

2. Stir together to make sure all ingredients have melted completely before removing from heat, then add essential oil drops.

3. Transfer mixture into an airtight container for storage. This recipe should fill about a ¼th jar if using a small container that comes with pump dispensers available at health food stores.

4. Apply face balm by massaging it onto your entire face, avoiding the eye area, then gently rub any excess on your neck until fully absorbed. You can use circular motions or patting motions, whatever feels most comfortable for you!

5. Wash off with water and pat dry. Exfoliate with a soft washcloth to remove dead skin cells, which will make your pores appear smaller over time!

You can make various balms at home with organic ingredients to suit your skin type and keep them in the fridge for a cool refreshing treat! We hope you've enjoyed this chapter about the benefits of organic lotions and balms. If it sounds like something that would work for your skin type, try out one or more recipes to see if they provide relief! You may find that balancing your hormones with natural remedies is a great way to promote healthy aging in other aspects of your life.

Chapter 8: Labeling and Gifting Your Goodies

As we get closer and closer to the end of our 10-part series, we will be discussing how you can label and gift your goodies. Labeling and gifting is a really important step in the process because it allows your customers to feel confident that they are purchasing from a reputable brand. Many people believe that by creating their products at home, there is no need for labeling or gifting. This couldn't be further from the truth! In this chapter, we'll be looking at how to store and label your finished products, as well as the importance of gifting them in lovely packaging.

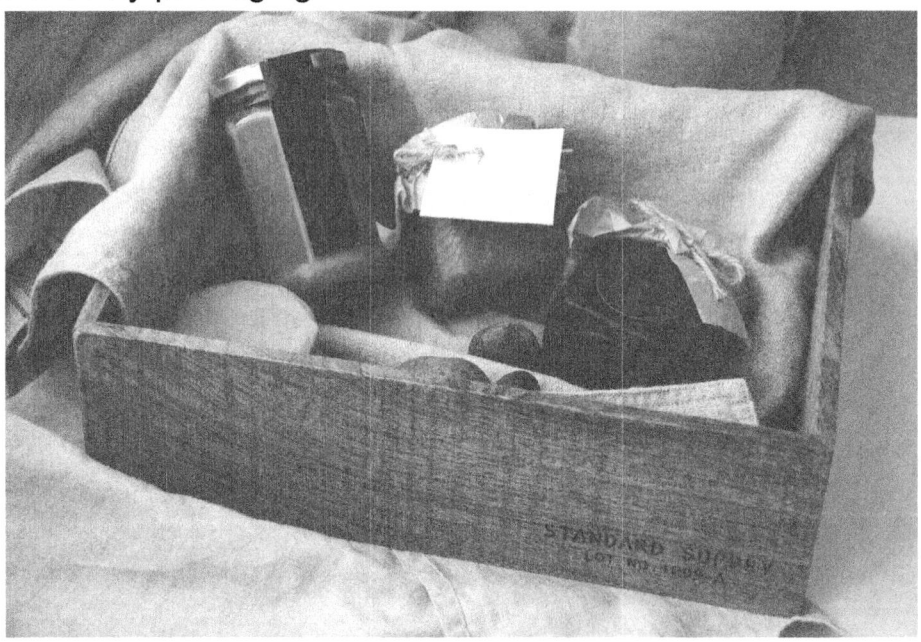

It is important to note that when you are making your skincare products at home, labeling and gifting of these goodies should be done correctly. This chapter will cover how to store, package, and label finished homemade skincare products. We will also discuss which containers should be used for each product and how to package them. Lastly, we will go over how to label the products with examples so that you can get your business off the ground without any legal issues or worries!

Choosing the Container Material

Many different materials can be used to package homemade cosmetics, but not all of them work well. Here is a list of the most common material types and their pros and cons:

Plastic

Plastic is the most common material used for packaging. It's cheap, lightweight, and very versatile; however, it can sometimes hold onto smells that could compromise your product or transfer to other products in storage.

The grade of plastic is important when looking for a container. The lower the grade, in general, the more harmful chemicals it will contain, which could leech into your products if not properly sealed.

Glass

Provided the glass has been properly sterilized before use, this is a great choice for packaging your products. In addition, there are many different types of jars that can be used with all sorts of lids available on the market today. However, regular Mason jar lids are the most common.

Metal

While metal is a great choice for product packaging, it does pose some problems. If you are looking at creating larger batches of your products that will be used at once or over multiple days, this may not be the best option because the metal can corrode and leak chemicals into your products if left unsealed for too long.

Ceramic

Ceramic is another great choice for product packaging. However, it can be expensive and cumbersome. Ceramic jars are usually used in smaller batches of products that will only last a few days or weeks at most.

Cork

Cork is a natural material that can be used to seal bottles. It is inexpensive and lasts for years without any harmful chemical leaching into your products. However, it must be kept wet, so if you live in an area where temperatures are very high or low, this may not work well for you.

Cork is a good alternative to glass if you are making candles, bath salts, or scrubs. However, it isn't suitable for creams, lotions, and balms because the pores in the cork allow bacteria to grow inside them.

Wood

Wood is the most common type of packaging for bath salts, candles, and scrubs. It isn't suitable for creams or lotions because it allows bacteria to grow inside it and spoils quickly when in contact with water. However, special types of wax can be used to coat wooden containers before use, preventing this.

Paper

Paper packaging is best for solid products like powders and salts. However, it isn't recommended for creams, lotions, or gels because they will dry out inside the package.

Cotton muslin bags are often used to store bath salts, scrubs, and loose teas. However, these aren't suitable to be used directly with the skin because they are porous and can harbor bacteria.

The most important thing to consider when choosing which container material you should use is whether or not it will keep out air, water, and other contaminants that could kill your skincare products before their shelf life has expired.

Here are a few important considerations for the storage of homemade products:

How to Store Homemade Cosmetics

When you package your homemade skincare products, it is important to store them somewhere that will not damage their ingredients or effectiveness. For example, if cooling and heating elements are constantly introduced into a product like an aloe vera gel (which loves room temperature), the living enzymes in the aloe vera gel could be killed off over time which would render the product useless.

The same can be said for products that need to remain in a cold environment, like creams and lotions, which are made with raw honey or Shea butter. If these types of containers are placed on top of or near heating elements, they could melt altogether over time! This is why it's so important to store your homemade cosmetics in the right place.

Cleanliness of Containers

Containers must be cleaned of any dirt or bacteria, which can cause the product to go bad over time. If you package your products in dirty containers without washing them first, this could introduce harmful microorganisms into your final goods.

If you are storing your cosmetics in plastic or glass jars, it is important to ensure that the packaging has been sterilized before use. This ensures that no harmful microorganisms have entered into the final product and compromised its effectiveness. Using a dishwasher and an oven will ensure that all of your containers are properly sterilized.

Light Exposure

Most homemade skincare products prefer to be stored in a cool, dark place, out of direct sunlight. This prevents the living enzymes from being killed off by exposure to UV light. If you are making creams or lotions using raw honey or Shea butter, these must remain sealed tightly away from any form of moisture, including humidity caused by room temperature, to avoid the growth of mold.

Knowing the Shelf Life of Your Homemade Cosmetics

The shelf life of your beauty products is determined by their ingredients, container type, and how they are stored.

Products that are water-based have a shorter shelf life than oil-based products because the latter can be preserved with vitamin E.

If you are making organic products that will be sold in a hot climate, the shelf life of your cosmetics is greatly reduced. This means that you should keep track of how long it's been since your product was made and always label them with expiration dates on every container to avoid any legal issues with customers who may have an allergic reaction or experience other side effects from using products which are past their prime.

Make to Order

This means that you should make your products as they are ordered. This ensures the freshest possible product is delivered to customers, preventing any legal issues with expired goods or compromised effectiveness caused by poor storage conditions over time.

Refrigeration and Freezing of Cosmetics

Some products – like aloe vera gel and castile soap – can be frozen, which helps to preserve them for longer periods. This is because many ingredients in homemade cosmetics do not have a very long shelf life.

Other products such as lotions and creams must remain refrigerated at all times as otherwise, they will melt. If you are making any products that must be refrigerated, it is important to inform your customers of this fact so they can store them in the right place at home.

Use Natural Preservatives

When making your own products, it is important to use natural preservatives when necessary. This will help preserve them for a longer period and prevent the growth of bacteria that can cause a product to go off over time if not correctly stored in the right conditions.

There are many different plant-based ingredients you can use as a natural preservative. These include grapefruit seed extract, rosemary oil, peppermint oil, and tea tree oil.

Packaging of Homemade Products for Retail

When customizing your packaging for your homemade cosmetics, you should take a few different factors into account.

Label Information

It is important to ensure that the labels on all of your products include an expiration date and instructions on how they should be used and what precautions need to be taken, if any.

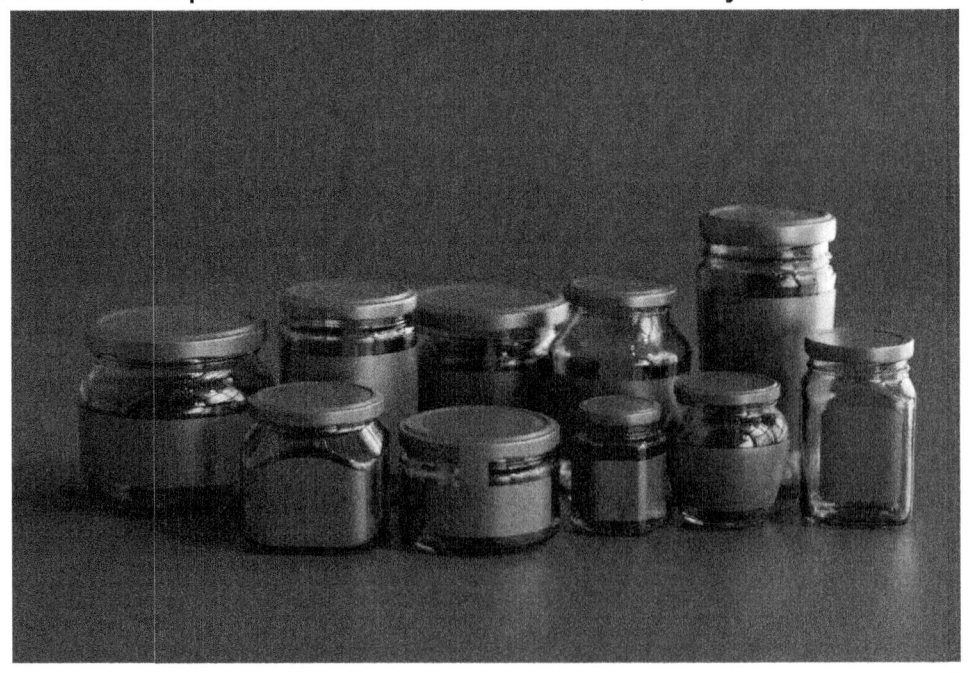

In addition, some ingredients may need to be kept away from direct sunlight, moisture, or heat, and this should all be included on the ingredients label. This information can also go into your product description for customers who are ordering online.

Finally, it is important that you clearly identify whether each item includes any animal-derived products like milk or honey, as well as which preservatives have been used.

All of these details should be included on your product label and in any other necessary places online to help customers make an informed decision about their purchase before they buy.

It is also important to list all the ingredients on the label, so customers know exactly what they are getting and can avoid potential allergic reactions.

Reusable or Recyclable Packaging?

When deciding how to package your homemade products, you should ask yourself whether they will be reusable or recyclable once a customer has finished using them.

If a product will be used up quickly, it makes sense to use packaging that can serve as the actual container for your cosmetics.

However, if you think that customers would prefer throwaway containers, this should be reflected in how you package them. In either case, make sure they are clearly labeled so there is no confusion regarding usage or the date when their guaranteed lifespan expires.

And, of course, the label should contain all the required information about how long an item has been open and when it needs to be discarded so that customers to use your products safely.

Identify Your Customer

Once you have started marketing your products, it is important to identify potential customers based on their needs.

Your packing should connect with your customer base in ways that are relevant to them.

For example, if you know your customers tend to be outdoorsy types who enjoy hiking and camping, then a rugged design is more likely to appeal to them than a sleek or fancy one.

When it comes down to deciding on the right aesthetics for your products, remember all the factors involved with selling them and how they will be used.

Designing Your Packaging for Homemade Products

When deciding on packaging designs, there are a few options to consider depending on whether you want an elegant or rustic design as well as the type of product you are making.

If your products include lotions and creams with light fragrances, it makes sense to create more minimalistic designs with clean lines.

On the other hand, if your product is something like soap or sunscreen with a strong scent and appearance, you should opt for simple packaging without too many colors or embellishments.

When designing labels for homemade products, keep in mind that they should be done in a way that is not too flashy or garish.

A good product design will highlight the key elements of your homemade item while still making it easy to read and understand what people are purchasing.

Remember, there are many ways you can customize your packaging, but you should make sure that whatever designs you choose should reflect your customer base and what they are looking for.

Identify Your Competition

Whether you have just created your first batch of handmade products or have been selling them for years, it is important to identify your competition in the industry. Whether they are small businesses or large corporations, knowing who else is out there doing similar work can help you make informed decisions about how to market your own products.

When you identify the competition, it is important to look at their branding and see what they are offering in terms of price and quality. By doing this research into other companies, you will be able to create a product with its own unique identity while still appealing to customers looking for similar things.

Pay Attention to the Weight of the Package

When designing the packaging for your product, it is important to keep in mind how much things weigh.

Postage charges for heavier packages can add up quickly, which means you will need to either charge more for your products or spend a lot on postage.

International Cosmetics Laws

When sending your products to customers in different countries, it is important to know what laws and regulations are applicable to cosmetics.

Different countries have their own rules about ingredients that can be used as well as whether or not you need a license to sell certain items.

A good way of finding this information is by contacting the country's government or checking on their website.

Canada

According to Health Canada's website, the federal department responsible for assisting Canadians to maintain and enhance their health analyzes cosmetic chemicals' safety. It prohibits or restricts the use of chemicals that pose a danger to people's health.

The Canadian government maintains a Cosmetic Ingredient Hotlist that includes hundreds of chemicals and pollutants that are prohibited or restricted to use in cosmetics, such as triclosan, nitrosamines, selenium, formaldehyde, and 1-4-dioxane.

Furthermore, cosmetic companies are not permitted to sell products that include hazardous chemicals, and you must disclose all cosmetic ingredients to Health Canada and must also register your goods with the government.

Europe

The European Union, which has grown to include 28 member states, has more strict and protective rules for cosmetics than the United States. Regardless of the chemical concentration, the EU Risk-Based Precautionary approach acknowledges that chemicals linked to cancer and congenital disabilities should not be used in cosmetics.

The European Union's safety directive prohibits the sale of 1,328 dangerous chemicals in cosmetics known or suspected to cause cancer, genetic damage, reproductive harm, or congenital disabilities.

The EU Cosmetics Directive protects the safety of cosmetic products by requiring pre-market safety evaluations, mandating cosmetic product registration, and authorizing the use of nanomaterials. Testing on animals is prohibited under EU law.

United States

The Federal Food, Drug, and Cosmetic Act (FD&C Act) and the Fair Packaging and Labeling Act (FPLA) are the two most essential cosmetic regulations in the United States.

Cosmetic products and components are not subject to premarket FDA approval under these statutes, with the exception of color additives. However, the promotion and sale of adulterated or misbranded cosmetics are unlawful.

The FDA has regulations that prohibit or restrict the use of specific hazard components in cosmetics (for example, Chloroform, mercuric compounds, and other chemicals on the list).

A cosmetic firm is free to utilize any substance as long as it is deemed safe for the intended usage.

Conducting Research to Understand Legal Regulations

Now that you have an idea of how important it is to be aware of legal regulations, the next step before creating your products would be to research what laws and regulations are applicable for cosmetics. It will save time, money, and frustration in the long run if product designs meet all requirements from each country they are being shipped out to.

Cosmetic manufacturing and the laws that govern it often vary from one country to another. To be successful in this industry, you must know what rules can affect your products and be aware of changes. In this chapter, we discussed how to store and package your homemade skincare products. Labeling is also very important because it lets the customer know what they're buying and if there are any side effects associated with that product. Always write the expiration date or manufacturing date so you don't accidentally sell a sour batch of lotion. Research the laws of your country to make sure you're not breaking any rules when selling products. Make sure you stay safe and follow all regulations.

Chapter 9: Ingredients Dictionary

Organic oils and ingredients are used in different recipes for homemade cosmetics. This can be difficult to keep up with, especially if you have a lot of recipes. That is why we created this list of organic ingredients and their corresponding oils!

List of Oils and Their Uses

Here is a list of the oils used in this book. This makes it easier to read and understand when looking for an oil that will work with your homemade recipe.

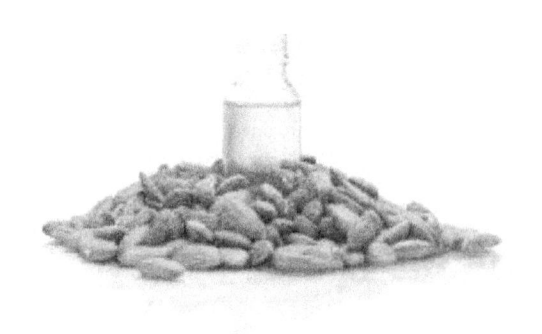

Almond Oil

Almond oil is a great oil to use when making homemade recipes. It is a lightweight oil that absorbs quickly and has many benefits for the skin, such as preventing acne. It can help prevent UV damage to the skin and reduce the appearance of scars. It also has a high vitamin E, A, B, D content, which is great for your skin.

Apricot Kernel Oil

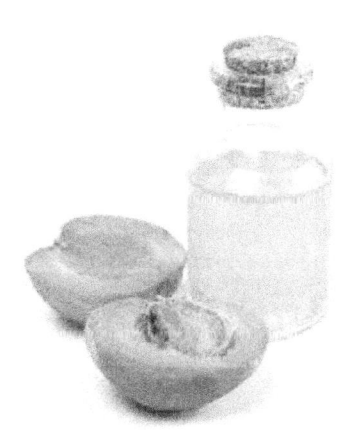

Apricot Kernel Oil is a lightweight oil that absorbs quickly, leaving the skin feeling smooth and soft. It's great for all skin types, especially dry or sensitive skin types, because it can soothe inflammation while being very gentle on the face. Apricot kernel oil is also rich in vitamin E. It is an antioxidant that helps the skin stay protected, leading to better-looking skin.

Argan Oil

Argan oil is a luxurious oil that has been used for centuries as an ingredient in beauty products. It's great to use on the skin and face because it absorbs quickly, leaving no greasy residue behind. Argan oil is high in linoleic and oleic fatty acids, two fats that are beneficial to health. It is also rich in vitamin E.

Avocado Oil

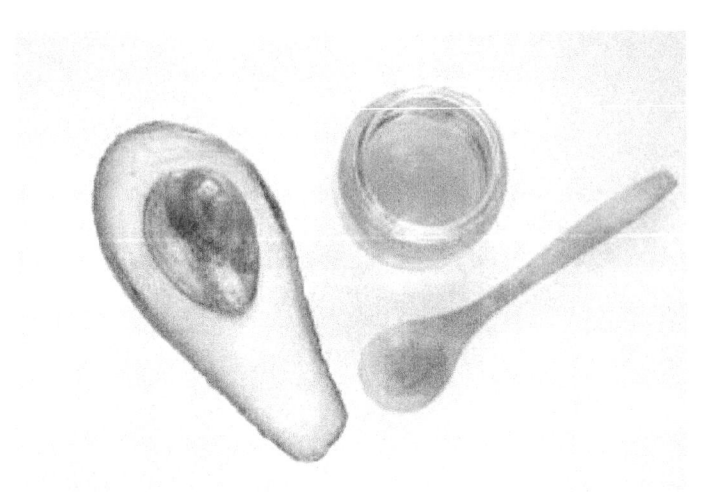

Avocado oil is a thick oil that absorbs slowly into the skin for nourishing benefits. It contains vitamins A, D, E, and lecithin, making it great for dry or aging skin. It is also great for sensitive, irritated, or red areas of the face (or anywhere on the body). Avocado oil has anti-inflammatory properties that help reduce pain and swelling in injured or damaged skin tissue.

Coconut Oil

Coconut oil can be used on the skin to moisturize, protect against sun damage, and reduce signs of aging over time. Coconut oil's inflammation-reducing and antibacterial qualities, as well as its components, may help with acne. Coconut oil contains antioxidants that fight free radicals in your body before they do any harm, such as attacking healthy cells and causing diseases. It also contains caprylic acid, lauric acid, and capric acid, all of which have antimicrobial properties that fight bad bacteria on the surface of your skin to prevent acne breakouts!

Chamomile Oil

Chamomile oil can reduce irritation, redness, and inflammation. It contains a compound called bisabolol that has anti-inflammatory properties to help soothe skin conditions such as eczema or psoriasis. Chamomile oil also has antibacterial qualities which fight acne-causing bacteria on the surface of your face.

Frankincense Oil

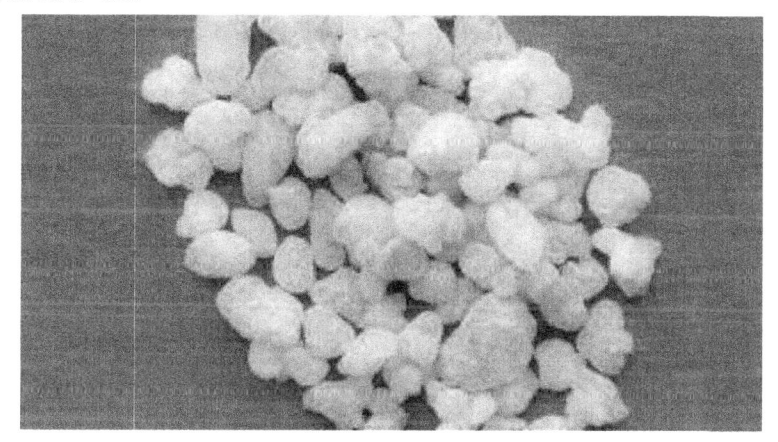

Frankincense oil is known for its anti-inflammatory properties, making it great to use on the face. It's also a source of antioxidants and antibacterial agents, making it perfect for fighting acne breakouts and minimizing existing scarring. Frankincense oil is a skin-friendly astringent. This implies that it can be used to treat blemishes and sores on the skin and other problems. As a healing oil, frankincense has long been recognized for repairing damaged skin. It is also beneficial for the reduction of stretch marks and scars.

Geranium Oil

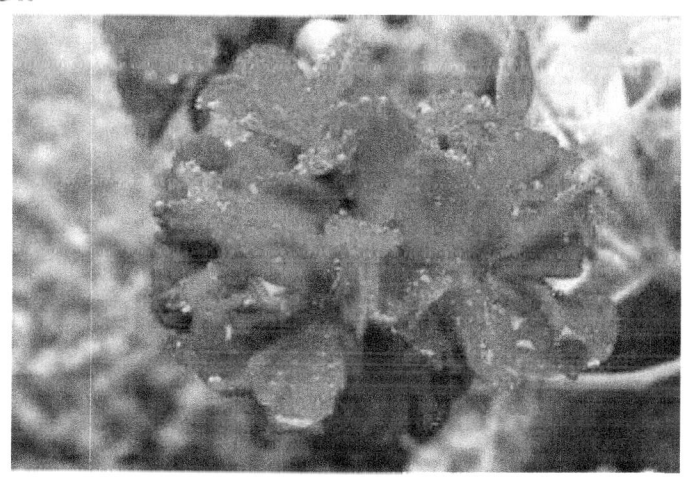

Geranium oil is a great moisturizer. It fights acne, eczema, or psoriasis while also softening dry patches of skin. This oil has anti-inflammatory properties to reduce redness and irritation and help minimize pain and swelling in case of rashes, infections, wounds, etc.

Grapeseed Oil

Grapefruit Seed Extract provides a low dose of antioxidants to your skin. It is a lightweight oil that absorbs quickly and can help with skin conditions such as acne, eczema, psoriasis, or dermatitis because it has anti-inflammatory properties which reduce the redness in these inflammatory skin disorders and leave your face feeling refreshed. It is also a source of Vitamin E.

Hazelnut Oil

Hazelnut oil has tannins in it, which are highly beneficial antioxidants. Tannins act as an astringent that may assist dry, greasy skin, cleanse, shrink pores, and remove harmful bacteria. This oil is known for its anti-inflammatory abilities to reduce the redness, irritation, or inflammation on your face! It has a high vitamin E and A content, which helps nourish dry patches of skin while softening it at the same time.

Jojoba Oil

Jojoba oil has been used for centuries as a moisturizer. It is great to use on the face because it contains anti-inflammatory properties which reduce redness and irritation while also helping to prevent acne breakouts. Jojoba oil can be applied directly onto dry skin areas such as elbows or knees. It will absorb into the skin quickly, leaving no greasy residue behind.

Lavender Oil

Lavender also has a variety of medicinal purposes. The micronutrients in this oil are vitamin B12, D, E, Copper, Selenium, Magnesium, and Zinc. Lavender oil can be used to fight acne, eczema, psoriasis, or dermatitis. It also has anti-inflammatory properties that help reduce pain and swelling in injured or damaged skin tissue. This oil is known for its calming effects, which can help reduce stress and anxiety.

Rose Oil

Rose oil is great for treating dry skin since it has many vitamins, antioxidants, and minerals. It also contains astringent components, making it an excellent acne fighter and redness and irritation reduction.

Rosehip Oil

Rosehip oil is filled with antioxidants and fatty acids. It's great for dry or irritated skin, as it can soothe inflammation while being very gentle on the face. Rosehip oil has a high concentration of vitamin A that helps stimulate collagen production to give firmer, more youthful-looking skin. This oil also contains omega-rich fatty acids and vitamin C and A. It also contains essential fatty acids such as gamma-linolenic acid, palmitic acid, oleic acid, and linoleic acid.

Vitamin F, a fatty acid made of linoleic acid and alpha-linolenic acid, is also present in rosehip oil.

All Other Ingredients
Aloe Vera
Aloe vera contains a variety of biologically active chemicals which include vitamins B2, B6, B1, C, niacinamide, glycoprotein enzymes, choline, phenolic compounds, phytochemicals, various amino acids, and salicylic acids.

Aloe vera helps to reduce inflammation, speeds up wound healing, and has anti-inflammatory properties to reduce the redness of inflamed skin tissue such as acne or rashes. It also contains antibacterial and antifungal agents, which can help prevent infections when applied topically onto areas affected by acne breakouts!

Apple Cider Vinegar
Apple cider vinegar contains various vitamins and minerals such as acetic acid, potassium, magnesium, calcium, vitamin A, C, and B-complex. It also has enzymes that aid in digestion while reducing inflammation to give your skin a healthy glow. Apple cider vinegar can be used on the face in place of chemical toners known for their harmful effects. It can help reduce the appearance of acne scars, wrinkles, and fine lines while evening out your skin tone to give it a healthy glow!

Bentonite Clay

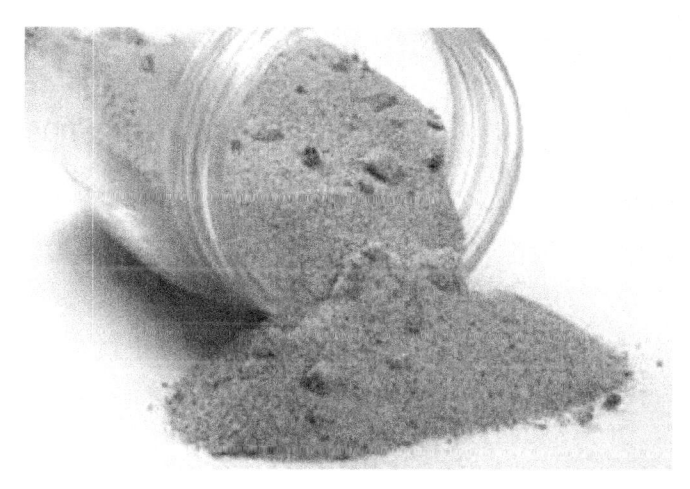

Bentonite clay contains a variety of minerals that are great for your skin. This includes calcium, magnesium, silica, sodium potassium, and iron. It also has antimicrobial components which help fight acne-causing bacteria while removing dead skin cells to give you an even complexion. Bentonite clay can be used on the face in place of chemical face masks, which are filled with harmful ingredients. It can help reduce the appearance of acne scars, wrinkles, and fine lines while evening out your skin tone to give it a healthy glow.

Charcoal Powder

This is a great ingredient for acne-prone skin. It has been used to treat and prevent breakouts as well as even out the complexion, reduce excess oil production, cleanse pores from dirt and other debris that may contribute to outbreaks. This powder also helps pull impurities from clogged pores, which prevent future blemishes from forming. It is helpful for people with oily skin as it reduces the appearance of oil production over time and also helps to reduce acne scars that may be left behind after healing. Charcoal powder can be added to facial masks, cleansers, or spot treatments to reap its benefits on the face and body.

Cocoa Powder

Cocoa powder is an excellent ingredient for dry, dull skin as it helps to brighten the complexion and give some life back to tired-looking skin. It contains antioxidants that help fight free radical damage caused by environmental elements such as pollution or UV rays, leading to early signs of aging like wrinkles and fine lines. It is a great source of bioactive phyto-compounds (epicatechin, catechin, and procyanidins), essential minerals magnesium and potassium), omega 3, vitamin E, fatty acids, and theobromine.

Glycerin

This ingredient is a humectant; it retains water and helps keep the skin hydrated. It also draws moisture from the air and traps it into your pores for prolonged benefits that can help prevent dryness or flaking, which may lead to irritation or itchiness. The best thing about glycerin? It's gentle enough even for those with sensitive skin.

Green Tea Extract

This ingredient is a natural antioxidant that has anti-inflammatory properties. It also contains bioactive compounds called polyphenols which are great for protecting against free radical damage and boosting the production of collagen in your skin, both of which help fight signs of aging like fine lines. Green tea extract can be used to treat acne since it helps control excess oil production and inflammation.

Rose Water

This water is a great source of vitamin C, which helps to brighten the complexion, keeping it looking fresh, youthful, and radiant. It also has anti-inflammatory properties that help soothe skin irritation such as redness or itchiness without drying out your skin, as many alcohol-based toners can do. Rosewater can be used to treat acne since it has anti-inflammatory properties that reduce redness and inflammation.

Olive Oil

This oil is great for those with dry, flaky skin. It acts like an emollient that helps smooth out the texture of your skin while also protecting against free radical damage caused by environmental elements such as pollution or UV rays.

Shea Butter

This ingredient is a great source of fatty acids and vitamin E, which help moisturize dry skin, looking smoother and more radiant. It's also been shown to be helpful for those with eczema as the fatty acids found in shea butter have anti-inflammatory properties that help calm the skin and reduce itchiness.

Turmeric

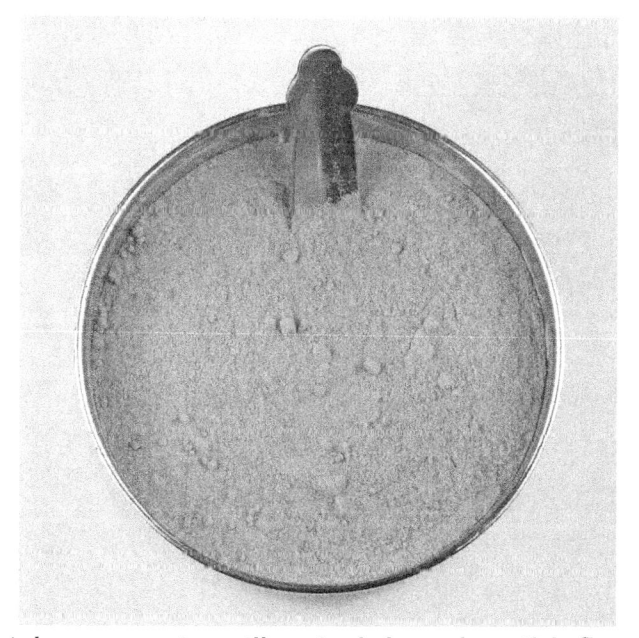

This ingredient is a great antibacterial and anti-inflammatory spice that can be applied topically to treat acne. It contains curcumin, which has been known to help lighten dark spots or pimple scars without damaging the skin like many harsh ingredients found in over-the-counter treatments do. It also has anti-aging benefits as it can help keep the skin looking and feeling smooth and firm.

Honey

This ingredient is a great source of antioxidants and antimicrobial properties that help fight free radical damage caused by environmental elements such as pollution or UV rays. Honey can also be used to treat acne since its antibacterial properties will kill off the bacteria that causes breakouts while moisturizing skin at the same time.

Honey is well-known for its skin benefits. It may help oily and acne-prone skin, thanks to its antibacterial and antiseptic properties. Honey is also a natural humectant, which keeps the skin moist without making it greasy. This is because humectants attract moisture from the skin without replacing it.

Skin Care Jargon, Explained

There is a lot of jargon used in the skincare industry, and it can be difficult to know what each ingredient does without doing a lot of research. Luckily, we've done most of that for you! Here is a summary of some popular buzzwords:

Antioxidants

These ingredients help fight free radical damage caused by environmental elements such as pollution or UV rays. They stop the oxidation of other molecules. Examples are Vitamin C, Vitamin E, and Green Tea Extract.

Humectants

These ingredients help draw moisture in from the air and trap it into your pores for prolonged benefits that can help prevent dryness or flaking, leading to irritation or itchiness. They're gentle enough, even for those with sensitive skin. Examples are Honey and Glycerin.

Emollients

These ingredients help smooth and soften the skin, making it look more radiant. This is especially helpful for those with dry or flaky skin who want to get rid of their flakes without turning to harsh chemicals that might irritate them instead. Examples are Olive oil and Shea Butter.

Anti-Inflammatory

This means an ingredient that reduces inflammation in your skin caused by breakouts or environmental factors such as pollution or UV rays. This is helpful for those with acne-prone skin who want to soothe redness and irritation without drying out their skin or irritating it further. Examples are Turmeric and Rosewater.

Preservatives

These ingredients help make your products last longer by inhibiting the growth of bacteria, yeast, fungi, etc., that could be harmful if they got into our product! The most common preservative is

Phenoxyethanol which has antimicrobial and anti-inflammatory benefits as well.

Antibacterial

This means an ingredient that reduces the growth of bacteria that could lead to acne or breakouts. This is helpful for those who want to fight off pimples naturally without turning to harsh chemicals found in over-the-counter treatments. Examples are Honey, Tea Tree Oil, Lavender Oil, and Salt.

Alcohol

This ingredient is used in toners, astringents, etc., to help reduce oil production by deeply cleansing the skin off pore-clogging dirt, sebum, or whatever else might be causing breakouts. It can also stop the growth of acne-causing bacteria because of its antibacterial properties. However, it can be very drying or irritating to the skin, so it is usually avoided in moisturizers.

Anti-Acne

This means an ingredient that reduces the growth of acne-causing bacteria on the surface of your skin without over-drying out your pores. This is helpful for those with oily and/or acne-prone skin who want to deeply cleanse without drying out their skin. Examples are Tea Tree Oil, Lavender Oil, and Salt.

Steroids

These ingredients reduce inflammation from acne or breakouts by reducing the overproduction of sebum that can clog pores and lead to pimple formation! They work best in spot treatments since if you use too much, it can cause thinning of the skin or other unwanted side effects. Examples are Salicylic Acid and Benzoyl Peroxide.

Retinol

This ingredient is a type of Vitamin A that acts as an antioxidant to protect against free radical damage, reduce signs of aging such as fine lines and wrinkles, fade post-acne marks and help prevent breakouts. It's a pretty powerful ingredient!

Alpha Hydroxy Acid

This organic acid derived from fruits helps remove the top layer of dead skin cells to reveal brighter, more even-toned, and refreshed-looking skin beneath. This can be especially helpful for those with oily or acne-prone skin as it helps to deeply cleanse without drying out. Examples are Glycolic Acid, Lactic Acid, and Citric Acid.

Niacinamide

This is a form of Vitamin B that helps fade post-acne marks and increase collagen production, which helps with signs of aging. It's especially helpful for those who want to reduce fine lines and wrinkles, fight off skin damage or fade post-acne marks.

Sebum

Sebum is the oily substance your skin naturally produces to keep it from drying out. This can be helpful as a moisturizer for those with dry or flaky skin, but if you have an oily T-zone and/or acne-prone skin, this ingredient could make things worse.

In this final chapter, we've explored the different ingredients and oils that are used in organic cosmetics. We hope you found it interesting to learn about how these natural ingredients can be combined with essential oils for various purposes.

Chapter 10: Skin Routine Planner

This chapter is about building an efficient skin care routine and organizing the recipes to add fun and variety. This chapter talks about why people should cleanse, moisturize every morning and night, what a skin care routine should look like, and in what order or time of the day each type of product should be applied. There is a detailed explanation of why you would want to use different products for your particular skin type, such as oily or dry skin. Finally, we will help you plan your monthly skin care routine.

What Is a Skin Care Routine?

Simply put: a skin care routine is a plan of how to care for your skin *every day.* It includes the type of products you use and in what order, and when to use them. A good starting point is to cleanse, tone, moisturize (and get into exfoliating, if needed) every day! In this chapter, we will go more in-depth on how to make your skin care routine efficient and effective.

Benefits of a Skin Care Routine

A skin care routine does a lot! Here are just some of the benefits:

Anti-Aging

A skin care routine can help reduce lines, wrinkles, and other signs of aging.

Hydration

A regular skin care routine keeps the skin hydrated, which helps it to stay healthy.

Treatment for Skin Conditions

If you have areas on your face that are dry or have redness, then a regular skin care routine will treat these conditions.

How to Build an Efficient Skin Care Routine

A skin care routine is a system of steps you follow to make your skin look its best. Without one, it can be tough (or even impossible) to get the results you want. A good regimen doesn't always need to include expensive products or hours in front of the mirror every day. In fact, sometimes *less is more.*

A typical skin care routine goes through a cycle of cleansing, toning, exfoliating, and moisturizing. Ideally, you should have a daytime routine for the morning and an evening routine to follow at night.

An ideal skin care regimen has a set of steps that are appropriate for your skin type, lifestyle requirements (like travel or exercise), and the weather conditions you live in. It's important to remember that one product may not work best in all areas; some products work better around the eyes, others on the cheeks, and so forth.

The first step of any skin care routine should be to look at your skin type (dry, oily, or combination) and what issues you're looking to fix, like acne breakouts or wrinkles. Once that is established, you can start building a routine around those needs.

Skin Care Routine for Oily Skin

If you have an oily skin type, the ideal goal is to take care of excess oil production and calm any inflammation or redness that results from it. You'll want a routine with gentle cleansers, toner, and moisturizer, as well as targeted treatments for breakouts such as spot treatment creams.

Step 1: Cleanse in the Morning and at Night

Cleansing your skin is the first step in any skin care routine. Most cleansers are gentle and work well on oily skin, but make sure you choose one that washes away without leaving a residue behind.

Look for ingredients like salicylic acid, glycolic or lactic acids to get your skin looking clear and feeling smooth.

Exfoliate once or twice a week with products containing small beads, which can help remove any buildup of dead skin cells.

Exfoliating and cleansing will help to prevent excess oil production while preventing dead skin cell buildup.

Step 2: Toning

Toners can also help close pores and tighten the skin, which keeps oil production in check. If you're looking for an extra-strong toner, look for products that contain salicylic acid, glycolic, or lactic acid.

Moisturizing should be left for last to seal in any skincare products before makeup application or environmental exposure. It's also a good practice to wait a few minutes after cleansing and applying toner so they both fully absorb into the skin.

Use a toner with anti-aging ingredients like vitamin C or retinol to keep your skin looking young and healthy over time. Do this every time you cleanse your skin.

Organic homemade toners like apple cider or rose water can also help with this.

Step 3: Treat Any Skin Ailments

Treating breakouts is the next step in your skin care routine if you have oily skin. Look for benzoyl peroxide or salicylic acid-based products to treat current acne outbreaks while preventing new ones from starting up.

To treat skin issues like large pores or blackheads, use clay masks that absorb excess oil while drawing out impurities.

Use this mask twice per week to help treat any skin ailments you have without over-drying the skin. Avoid using these more than twice per week, as they can dry out your skin over time.

Step 4: Moisturize in the Morning and at Night

Moisturizing is the final step of your skin care routine and should be done after cleansing and toning. Look for a moisturizer that works well with your skin type. If you have oily skin, look for lighter formulations containing gel, while those with dry skin will benefit from thicker creams and serums.

Organic homemade moisturizers like avocado oil, coconut cream, or shea butter can also help with this.

Other Important Steps for Oily Skin

It is also important to use sunscreen, as the skin on your face is most sensitive and prone to sun damage. Look for one with at least an SPF 30 that will protect against both UVA and UVB rays.

Use blotting paper to absorb excess oil throughout the day.

Apply a thin layer of mineral powder over your makeup if you need it to last longer, without smudging or caking up on oily skin types.

Skin Care Routine for Dry Skin

Dry skin is caused by a lack of natural oils, leaving skin feeling tight and itchy. Using harsh products that strip away the moisture in your skin will only cause more oil production to compensate for the dryness.

Dry skin could be a result of internal or external factors. With an efficient skin care routine, we will target to address the external factors.

Step 1: Cleansing

For dry skin types, use a hydrating cleanser. Cleansers with a creamy texture are best for dry skin, as they'll help to retain moisture after cleansing.

Cleansing is the first step in this routine because it's going to remove excess sebum and dead cells from your face without stripping away all-natural oils from your skin. Use an oil-based cleanser that will moisturize while cleaning.

Natural ingredients like rosehip oil, jojoba, and evening primrose are good options for dry skin.

Step 2: Toner

Toners with alcohol are too harsh for dry skin. Instead, use a toner that contains tea tree oil to help balance your skin's pH levels.

Step 3: Treatment for Dry Skin Ailments

Dry skin can lead to conditions like psoriasis. Treat dry skin by using a moisturizer that contains hyaluronic acid or glycerin, which will help your body retain moisture.

Anti-aging products for dry skin should contain ceramides, which help to strengthen the protective layer on your face and prevent further damage.

Step 4: Moisturizer with SPF

To protect your newly hydrated skin (and maintain a youthful look), use a moisturizer that contains sunscreen every day. Applying an anti-aging serum before moisturizing will also give you added benefits of more collagen production and prevent fine lines and wrinkles. This routine is perfect for those who have sensitive or acne-prone skin types as well!

For combination skin, use the same routine but change your products for specific areas.

For combination skin, follow steps one through three above, and then choose a moisturizer that is appropriate for either dry or oily spots on your face. The key to maintaining clear skin while also keeping it hydrated is by exfoliating regularly.

Importance of Cleansing and Moisturizing

Cleaning is one of the most critical steps in any skin care routine because it removes dirt, oil, and makeup that can clog pores.

Moisturizing keeps your skin hydrated by locking in moisture to prevent dryness or flaking. It also helps to protect against sun damage and premature aging. Make sure you choose a moisturizer that works with your type of skin! This doesn't have to be complicated; all it takes are three simple steps every day for clear, healthy-looking skin.

You must ideally cleanse and moisturize twice- in the am and the pm.

When to Use Skincare Products

It is important to know when and how to use skincare products, as some can do more harm than good if used incorrectly.

Cleansing

Use a gentle cleanser that is appropriate for your skin type twice daily. If you wear makeup, feel free to double cleanse by removing all the dirt and oil first with an oil-based product before cleansing again with a water-based one. Make sure not to over-dry your skin by using harsh scrubs or rough cloth on delicate facial tissue.

Toners

Toners allow deeper penetration of active ingredients within skincare products, such as Vitamin C and other antioxidants. These can be used for all skin types, but they may be too hard for dry skin if not properly moisturized.

Use a toner by applying it with a cotton pad. Gently wipe over your face and neck in upward strokes; try not to rub too harshly on areas such as around your eyes where the tissues are thinner and more susceptible to damage from rubbing.

Toners should be applied every time you wash your face or after you've removed makeup.

Moisturizer

Dry skin should use rich moisturizers, while oily or acne-prone skin types should strive to use light water-based ones. Apply your cream twice daily by gently patting it onto the face and neck with clean hands; concentrate on areas where you tend to lose more moisture, such as around your eyes, lips, cheeks, and forehead.

Face Creams

Face creams are ideal for all skin types, especially sensitive ones. They contain more active skincare ingredients than moisturizers and provide a barrier against environmental elements such as pollution or damaging UV rays, which can cause premature aging.

Apply face cream by gently patting it onto your face with clean hands after you've applied any serums or treatments to ensure they penetrate deep enough into your skin before adding another layer on top that might hinder the absorption rate.

Use it as a replacement for your moisturizer if your skin is on the oilier side, or use it in addition to a rich cream for dryer types.

Eye Cream

Apply a small amount of eye cream to the back of your ring finger with clean hands before gently rubbing it into the under-eye area and eyelids up towards your eyebrows. This is especially important for those who wear makeup during the day that can settle in fine lines, making them appear darker than they are.

Use while you are applying your moisturizer, typically in the morning and evening.

Sunscreen

Wear sunscreen every day, no matter which season it is or even if you're just sitting by a window that lets in UV rays. Most sunscreens will last an average of 30 minutes, so apply generously before heading out for an extended period of time.

Use at least 15-30 minutes before going outside to allow complete absorption into the skin. Reapply every two hours, when outdoors or more often, depending on how much exposure there is to the sun, such as swimming or exercise, which can make you sweat off some protection from sunscreen! However, it should be noted that products with physical blockers tend to sit better on the skin than chemical ones, but either one still needs to be reapplied if you're going in and out of the sun all day.

Serums/Ampoules/Masks

These products contain active ingredients like retinol or vitamin C but should be used sparingly by all skin types due to their potency. If you choose to use these, make sure not to overuse them (no more than twice per week) and to wait at least 30 minutes before applying anything else on top of them.

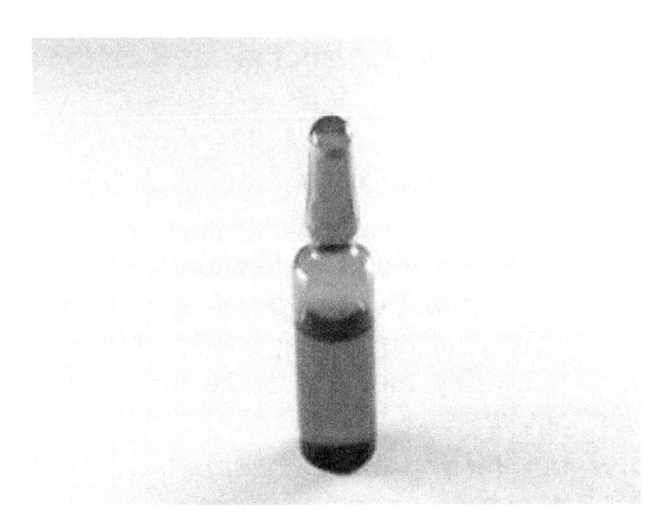

Product Type	Sunday	Monday	Tuesday	Wednesday	Thursday	Friday	Saturday
Cleanser							
Face Scrub							
Toner							
Face Cream							
Eye Cream							
Serum							
Moisturizer/ Lotion/ Body Butter							
Mask							
Face Balm							
Body Scrub							

Serums are best used in the morning after toning; ampoules/masks can be applied by all skin types once or twice a week, but not more than that, depending on how sensitive your skin is.

If you have dry skin, aim for serums instead, while those with oily skin should stick with masks or ampoules if they're looking for more hydration benefits from these products. And lastly, acne-prone skin types may benefit most from using both serum AND mask together daily because their active ingredients are so concentrated, which makes it easier to get rid of blemishes faster without over-drying the area.

Skin Care Routine Template for 30 Days

Here is a calendar with a 30-day layout that you can follow if you're looking for an easy way to organize your skin care routine.

Date	Product	AM	PM
1	Cleanser		
	Face Scrub		
	Toner		
	Face Cream		
	Eye Cream		
	Serum		
	Moisturizer/Lotion/Body Butter		
	Mask		
	Face Balm		
	Body Scrub		
2	Cleanser		
	Face Scrub		
	Toner		
	Face Cream		
	Eye Cream		
	Serum		
	Moisturizer/Lotion/Body Butter		
	Mask		
	Face Balm		
	Body Scrub		

3	Cleanser		
	Face Scrub		
	Toner		
	Face Cream		
	Eye Cream		
	Serum		
	Moisturizer/Lotion/Body Butter		
	Mask		
	Face Balm		
	Body Scrub		
4	Cleanser		
	Face Scrub		
	Toner		
	Face Cream		
	Eye Cream		
	Serum		
	Moisturizer/Lotion/Body Butter		
	Mask		
	Face Balm		
	Body Scrub		
5	Cleanser		
	Face Scrub		
	Toner		

	Face Cream		
	Eye Cream		
	Serum		
	Moisturizer/Lotion/Body Butter		
	Mask		
	Face Balm		
	Body Scrub		
6	Cleanser		
	Face Scrub		
	Toner		
	Face Cream		
	Eye Cream		
	Serum		
	Moisturizer/Lotion/Body Butter		
	Mask		
	Face Balm		
	Body Scrub		
7	Cleanser		
	Face Scrub		
	Toner		
	Face Cream		
	Eye Cream		
	Serum		

	Moisturizer/Lotion/Body Butter		
	Mask		
	Face Balm		
	Body Scrub		
8	Cleanser		
	Face Scrub		
	Toner		
	Face Cream		
	Eye Cream		
	Serum		
	Moisturizer/Lotion/Body Butter		
	Mask		
	Face Balm		
	Body Scrub		
9	Cleanser		
	Face Scrub		
	Toner		
	Face Cream		
	Eye Cream		
	Serum		
	Moisturizer/Lotion/Body Butter		
	Mask		
	Face Balm		

	Body Scrub		
10	Cleanser		
	Face Scrub		
	Toner		
	Face Cream		
	Eye Cream		
	Serum		
	Moisturizer/Lotion/Body Butter		
	Mask		
	Face Balm		
	Body Scrub		
11	Cleanser		
	Face Scrub		
	Toner		
	Face Cream		
	Eye Cream		
	Serum		
	Moisturizer/Lotion/Body Butter		
	Mask		
	Face Balm		
	Body Scrub		
12	Cleanser		
	Face Scrub		

	Toner		
	Face Cream		
	Eye Cream		
	Serum		
	Moisturizer/Lotion/Body Butter		
	Mask		
	Face Balm		
	Body Scrub		
13	Cleanser		
	Face Scrub		
	Toner		
	Face Cream		
	Eye Cream		
	Serum		
	Moisturizer/Lotion/Body Butter		
	Mask		
	Face Balm		
	Body Scrub		
14	Cleanser		
	Face Scrub		
	Toner		
	Face Cream		
	Eye Cream		

	Serum		
	Moisturizer/Lotion/Body Butter		
	Mask		
	Face Balm		
	Body Scrub		
15	Cleanser		
	Face Scrub		
	Toner		
	Face Cream		
	Eye Cream		
	Serum		
	Moisturizer/Lotion/Body Butter		
	Mask		
	Face Balm		
	Body Scrub		
16	Cleanser		
	Face Scrub		
	Toner		
	Face Cream		
	Eye Cream		
	Serum		
	Moisturizer/Lotion/Body Butter		
	Mask		

	Face Balm		
	Body Scrub		
17	Cleanser		
	Face Scrub		
	Toner		
	Face Cream		
	Eye Cream		
	Serum		
	Moisturizer/Lotion/Body Butter		
	Mask		
	Face Balm		
	Body Scrub		
18	Cleanser		
	Face Scrub		
	Toner		
	Face Cream		
	Eye Cream		
	Serum		
	Moisturizer/Lotion/Body Butter		
	Mask		
	Face Balm		
	Body Scrub		
19	Cleanser		

	Face Scrub		
	Toner		
	Face Cream		
	Eye Cream		
	Serum		
	Moisturizer/Lotion/Body Butter		
	Mask		
	Face Balm		
	Body Scrub		
20	Cleanser		
	Face Scrub		
	Toner		
	Face Cream		
	Eye Cream		
	Serum		
	Moisturizer/Lotion/Body Butter		
	Mask		
	Face Balm		
	Body Scrub		
21	Cleanser		
	Face Scrub		
	Toner		
	Face Cream		

		Eye Cream		
		Serum		
		Moisturizer/Lotion/Body Butter		
		Mask		
		Face Balm		
		Body Scrub		
22		Cleanser		
		Face Scrub		
		Toner		
		Face Cream		
		Eye Cream		
		Serum		
		Moisturizer/Lotion/Body Butter		
		Mask		
		Face Balm		
		Body Scrub		
23		Cleanser		
		Face Scrub		
		Toner		
		Face Cream		
		Eye Cream		
		Serum		
		Moisturizer/Lotion/Body Butter		

	Mask		
	Face Balm		
	Body Scrub		
24	Cleanser		
	Face Scrub		
	Toner		
	Face Cream		
	Eye Cream		
	Serum		
	Moisturizer/Lotion/Body Butter		
	Mask		
	Face Balm		
	Body Scrub		
25	Cleanser		
	Face Scrub		
	Toner		
	Face Cream		
	Eye Cream		
	Serum		
	Moisturizer/Lotion/Body Butter		
	Mask		
	Face Balm		
	Body Scrub		

26	Cleanser		
	Face Scrub		
	Toner		
	Face Cream		
	Eye Cream		
	Serum		
	Moisturizer/Lotion/Body Butter		
	Mask		
	Face Balm		
	Body Scrub		
27	Cleanser		
	Face Scrub		
	Toner		
	Face Cream		
	Eye Cream		
	Serum		
	Moisturizer/Lotion/Body Butter		
	Mask		
	Face Balm		
	Body Scrub		
28	Cleanser		
	Face Scrub		
	Toner		

	Face Cream		
	Eye Cream		
	Serum		
	Moisturizer/Lotion/Body Butter		
	Mask		
	Face Balm		
	Body Scrub		
29	Cleanser		
	Face Scrub		
	Toner		
	Face Cream		
	Eye Cream		
	Serum		
	Moisturizer/Lotion/Body Butter		
	Mask		
	Face Balm		
	Body Scrub		
30	Cleanser		
	Face Scrub		
	Toner		
	Face Cream		
	Eye Cream		
	Serum		

	Moisturizer/Lotion/Body Butter		
	Mask		
	Face Balm		
	Body Scrub		
31	Cleanser		
	Face Scrub		
	Toner		
	Face Cream		
	Eye Cream		
	Serum		
	Moisturizer/Lotion/Body Butter		
	Mask		
	Face Balm		
	Body Scrub		

If you've read this far, I hope that by now, you know more about how your skin operates and the importance of having a routine. A good skin care routine can be an investment of both time and money, but it will pay off with clearer, younger-looking skin! It may seem like there are too many steps involved in the process of taking care of your skin properly, but if we break this down into manageable chunks for each day (morning/night), then it won't feel so overwhelming anymore. And don't forget: The simplest routines work best because they're easier to maintain all year long. Don't give up on yourself or your goals just because things get difficult along the way! You have what it takes to be successful with your skin care; we believe in you!

Conclusion

Congratulations! You have reached the conclusion of this guide to making your natural skincare products.

In this book, we discussed the main ingredients used in skincare products, with information specific to each ingredient. We have gone over different types of products, including cleansers, moisturizers, scrubs, masks, serums, and balms. You should now be confident to make any or all of these items to use for yourself or friends and family.

We also discussed packaging and labeling, and hopefully, you have been inspired to get creative about how you can present your creations. Legal aspects of labeling and packaging were also discussed for those who wish to sell their goodies.

Finally, we went over a basic skin care routine that you can use as a template for your very own natural skin care regimen.

If you have been reading from start to finish, you should now be a pro at making your organic skincare goodies.

But don't stop! There are so many more ingredients to experiment with and yummy recipes to concoct. Keep on reading other natural beauty blogs, forums, and websites. Always stay informed, as a good skincare connoisseur should do. Be sure to read labels when shopping for new products too. Many "organic" moisturizers still contain nasty preservatives and skin-irritating chemicals that you should avoid.

Here are some helpful suggestions to keep in mind when making your natural beauty products:

- Be creative! Don't be afraid to experiment with different essential oils, carrier oils, herbs, flowers, or fruits. You can always mix things up until you find the perfect concoction.
- The more natural, the better! If you are using an oil in your recipes for its moisturizing benefits, try to stick to organic cold-

pressed oils. Also, think about making your carrier oils too.

- When crafting your goodies, keep notes of what works well together and what does not, so you can create your recipes or adapt the existing ones to your liking next time.
- Have fun!

That's it for this guide on how to make organic skincare products. I hope you enjoyed reading through the DIY packages and found some interesting tips and tricks to incorporate into your natural skin care routine. Remember, always keep things simple because too many ingredients can be too harsh on your skin, especially if you are new to making DIY goodies.

Making organic skincare products can be a fun experience. If you follow the recipes carefully and use all-natural ingredients, you should have no problem making your homemade body care products.

I hope you try out some of the recipes in this guide or come up with your own creations. Happy natural skin care!

Printed in Great Britain
by Amazon